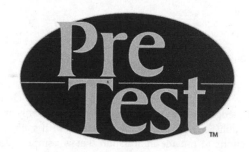

Family Medicine

PreTest™ Self-Assessment and Review

Notice

Medicine is an ever-changing science. As new research and clinical experience broaden our knowledge, changes in treatment and drug therapy are required. The authors and the publisher of this work have checked with sources believed to be reliable in their efforts to provide information that is complete and generally in accord with the standards accepted at the time of publication. However, in view of the possibility of human error or changes in medical sciences, neither the authors nor the publisher nor any other party who has been involved in the preparation or publication of this work warrants that the information contained herein is in every respect accurate or complete, and they disclaim all responsibility for any errors or omissions or for the results obtained from use of the information contained in this work. Readers are encouraged to confirm the information contained herein with other sources. For example and in particular, readers are advised to check the product information sheet included in the package of each drug they plan to administer to be certain that the information contained in this work is accurate and that changes have not been made in the recommended dose or in the contraindications for administration. This recommendation is of particular importance in connection with new or infrequently used drugs.

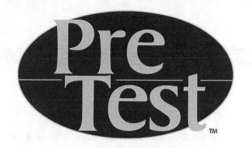

Family Medicine

PreTest™ Self-Assessment and Review

Second Edition

Doug Knutson, MD
Associate Professor, Family Medicine
Program Director, Family Medicine Residency
The Ohio State University
Columbus, Ohio

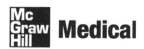

New York   Chicago   San Francisco   Lisbon   London   Madrid   Mexico City
Milan   New Delhi   San Juan   Seoul   Singapore   Sydney Toronto

Family Medicine: PreTest™ Self-Assessment and Review, Second Edition

Copyright © 2009, 2008 by the McGraw-Hill Companies, Inc. All rights reserved. Printed in the United States of America. Except as permitted under the United States Copyright Act of 1976, no part of this publication may be reproduced or distributed in any form or by any means, or stored in a database or retrieval system, without the prior written permission of the publisher.

PreTest™ is a trademark of the McGraw-Hill Companies, Inc.

1 2 3 4 5 6 7 8 9 0   DOC/DOC   12 11 10 9

ISBN 978-0-07-159888-0
MHID 0-07-159888-X

This book was set in Berkeley by International Typesetting and Composition.
The editors were Kirsten Funk and Peter J. Boyle.
The production supervisor was Sherri Souffrance.
Project management was provided by Harleen Chopra, International Typesetting and
    Composition.
RR Donnelley was printer and binder.

This book is printed on acid-free paper.

Library of Congress Cataloging-in-Publication Data

Knutson, Doug (Douglas J.), 1962-
    Family medicine : PreTest self-assessment and review / Doug Knutson.
— 2nd ed.
        p. ; cm.
    Includes bibliographical references and index.
    ISBN-13: 978-0-07-159888-0 (pbk. : alk. paper)
    ISBN-10: 0-07-159888-X (alk. paper)
    1. Family medicine—Examinations, questions, etc.   I. Title.
    [DNLM: 1. Family Practice—Examination Questions. WB 18.2 K67f   2009]
    RC58.K58   2009
    616—dc22   2008052991

Student Reviewers

Lindsay K. Botsford, MD
Baylor University
Kelsey-Seybold Family Medicine Residency Program
PGY-2

Joshua Lynch
Lake Erie College of Osteopathic Medicine
Class of 2008

Amanda B. Sosulski
SUNY Upstate Medical University
Class of 2009

Kevyn To
SUNY Upstate Medical University
Class of 2009

Contents

Acknowledgments

Special thanks to Cari Brackett, PharmD, for her help with questions and references, Gina Stevens for her support and never ending positivity, the Ohio State University medical students and Family Medicine residents for inspiring me to be a better teacher, the OSU Department of Family Medicine for the developmental opportunities afforded to me, and, most importantly, John and Lucy for their support and encouragement.

Introduction

Family Medicine: PreTest™ Self Assessment and Review, Second Edition, is intended to provide medical students, as well as house officers and physicians, with a convenient tool for assessing and improving their knowledge of medicine. The 500 questions in this book are similar in format and complexity to those included in Step 2 of the United States Medical Licensing Examination (USMLE). They may also be a useful study tool for Step 3.

For multiple-choice questions, the *one best* response to each question should be selected. For matching sets, a group of questions will be preceded by a list of lettered options. For each question in the matching set, select *one* lettered option that is *most* closely associated with the question. Each question in this book has a corresponding answer, a reference to a text that provides background to the answer, and a short discussion of various issues raised by the question and its answer. A listing of references for the entire book follows the last chapter.

To simulate the time constraints imposed by the qualifying examinations for which this book is intended as a practice guide, the student or physician should allot about 1 minute for each question. After answering all questions in a chapter, as much time as necessary should be spent in reviewing the explanations for each question at the end of the chapter. Attention should be given to all explanations, even if the examinee answered the question correctly. Those seeking more information on a subject should refer to the reference materials listed or to other standard texts in medicine.

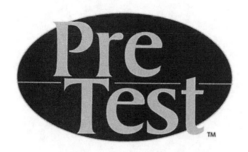

Family Medicine

PreTest™ Self-Assessment and Review

Preventive Medicine

Questions

Immunizations

1. You are examining a normal-term newborn whose mother is hepatitis B virus surface antigen positive. Which of the following protocols is recommended for the child?

   a. Hepatitis B vaccination at 0 to 2 months, a second dose at 1 to 4 months, and a third dose at 6 to 18 months of age
   b. Hepatitis B vaccination within 12 hours of birth, with the timing of the second and third doses based on the mother's hepatitis B viral load at the time of delivery
   c. Hepatitis B vaccination and hepatitis B immune globulin within 12 hours of birth, a second dose of hepatitis B vaccine at 1 to 2 months, and a third dose of vaccine at 6 months
   d. Hepatitis B vaccination and hepatitis B immune globulin within 12 hours of birth, a second dose of the vaccine and immune globulin at 1 to 2 months, and a third dose of the vaccine and immune globulin at 6 months
   e. Hepatitis B vaccination at birth, with serologic testing of the baby before additional vaccinations are given

2. You are counseling a mother about her child's immunization schedule. She asks specifically if her child would benefit from the *Haemophilus influenzae* type b (Hib) vaccine. Which of the following statements is true about this vaccine?

   a. The vaccine is between 95% to 100% effective in preventing invasive Hib disease.
   b. The vaccine will help to prevent otitis media caused by *H influenzae*.
   c. Adverse reactions to the vaccine include an unusual high-pitched cry, high fevers, and seizures.
   d. The first vaccine should be administered at birth.
   e. The vaccine cannot be given concurrently with other vaccines.

✓ **3.** You are discussing varicella-zoster vaccination with a 34-year-old man who does not ever remember having chicken pox. Which of the following statements is true?

a. Varicella-zoster infection is less severe in adults.
b. Two doses of the vaccine are required, 4 to 8 weeks apart.
c. Serologic testing for varicella antibodies is necessary before vaccination.
d. If the patient lives with an immunocompromised person, vaccination should be avoided.
e. The subsequent risk of zoster is higher among those who have been vaccinated as compared with those who had natural infection.

4. An elderly patient that you follow has recently started volunteering at a hospital and requires hepatitis B vaccination. You find that he is hepatitis B surface antibody positive. Which of the following would be the best guideline to follow in this case?

a. No vaccination is necessary based on his laboratory evaluation.
b. Administer one dose of hepatitis B vaccine.
c. Administer two doses of hepatitis B vaccine, at least 1 month apart.
d. Administer two doses of hepatitis B vaccine, at least 6 months apart.
e. Administer three does of hepatitis B vaccine at the appropriate time interval.

5. You are caring for a 23-year-old healthy homosexual male who works as an accountant and lives alone. He had the "typical childhood vaccinations" and provides documentation of his immunization record. He is up to date on tetanus, and was primarily immunized against diphtheria, pertussis, polio, hepatitis B, measles, mumps, rubella, and *H influenzae* type b. Which of the following vaccinations is indicated for this patient?

a. Varicella
b. Meningococcus
c. Hepatitis A
d. Pneumococcus
e. A booster of the measles-mumps-rubella (MMR) vaccine

6. In the prenatal workup for a 24-year-old patient, you discover she is not immune to rubella. When is the best time to vaccinate her against rubella?

a. Immediately
b. In the second trimester of pregnancy
c. In the third trimester of pregnancy
d. In the early postpartum period
e. At least 4 weeks postpartum

7. A 32-year-old woman comes to your office for a complete physical examination. When discussing her vaccinations, you discover that she received her primary tetanus series as a child, and her last tetanus booster was 11 years ago. Which of the following is true?

a. No vaccination is required.
b. The patient should receive a tetanus-diphtheria (Td) booster.
c. The patient should receive tetanus immune globulin.
d. The patient should receive a diphtheria-tetanus-pertussis (DTP) immunization.
e. The patient should receive tetanus, diphtheria, and acellular pertussis (Tdap) immunization.

8. You are caring for a woman who would like her children vaccinated against influenza. Her children are ages 4 months, 24 months, and 5 years. Which of the following represents current immunization recommendations for influenza?

a. None of her children should be vaccinated.
b. The 4-month-old and the 24-month-old should be vaccinated.
c. The 24-month-old and the 5-year-old should be vaccinated.
d. Only the 24-month-old should be vaccinated.
e. All the children should be vaccinated.

9. You are caring for a 2½-year-old boy who is coming to your office for the first time. Reviewing his immunization record, you find that he has never received vaccination for invasive pneumococcal disease using the 7-valent pneumococcal conjugate vaccine. Which of the following is true regarding recommendations in his case?

a. He is no longer at risk for invasive pneumococcal disease, and does not need to be vaccinated.
b. He should only be vaccinated if he has an immunocompromising condition.
c. He should only be vaccinated if he has a congenital or genetic pulmonary condition.
d. He should be vaccinated, and should start the usual series for primary vaccination.
e. He should be vaccinated, but with a modified schedule for immunization.

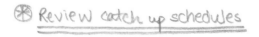 Review catch up schedules

10. You are caring for a 30-year-old woman who asks you about the human papillomavirus (HPV) vaccination. She is recently divorced and not in a monogamous relationship. She has a history of genital warts, and had an abnormal Papanicolaou (Pap) test 2 years ago, for which she underwent colposcopy, biopsy, and cryotherapy. Subsequent Pap tests have been normal. Which is the following is true?

a. She is unable to be vaccinated because she has a history of genital warts.
b. She is unable to be vaccinated because she has a history of an abnormal Pap test.
c. She is unable to be vaccinated because she is not in a monogamous relationship.
d. Vaccination is not recommended for 30-year-old women.
e. She should be vaccinated.

11. You are determining which of the patients in your practice should receive the quadrivalent HPV vaccination. This vaccine is inappropriate for which of the following patients?

a. An 18-year-old woman with an abnormal Pap test that has yet to be followed up appropriately.
b. A 16-year-old girl who recently delivered her first child and is currently breast-feeding.
c. A pregnant 14-year-old.
d. A 12-year-old with asthma currently taking steroids for an exacerbation.
e. An 11-year-old victim of sexual abuse.

12. A recently retired 67-year-old woman presents to you to establish care. She was a long time smoker, but quit 5 years ago. She is generally healthy, but her prior physician told her that she has "emphysema." She was prescribed an "inhaler" to use as-needed and only uses it rarely. She asks about necessary immunizations. Assuming she has not had the vaccine before, which of the following vaccines should she receive?

a. MMR
b. Tdap
c. Varicella
d. Pneumococcal polysaccharide
e. Intranasal influenza

13. Of the following, which patient would be considered the most appropriate candidate for vaccination against herpes zoster?

a. A 53-year-old man with a history of chicken pox as a child and a personal history of diabetes mellitus
b. A 58-year-old woman who recently underwent successful surgery for colon cancer
c. A 33-year-old man who was recently diagnosed with human immunodeficiency virus (HIV)
d. A 22-year-old with a personal history of sickle-cell disease
e. A 66-year-old man with a personal history of shingles at age 56

Screening Tests

14. You are discussing preventive health screening with a college student. He has no family history of hypertension, coronary artery disease, diabetes, or cancer. At what age should you consider screening for lipid disorders?

a. 18 years
b. 21 years
c. 25 years
d. 35 years
e. 50 years

15. You are seeing a 58-year-old smoker for a routine health examination. You have counseled him on discontinuing tobacco use, and he is considering that alternative. He denies coughing, shortness of breath, or hemoptysis. Which of the following is a recommended screen for lung cancer in this patient?

a. He should not be screened for lung cancer.
b. Chest x-ray.
c. Chest computed tomography (CT).
d. Sputum cytology.
e. Bronchoscopy.

16. You are seeing a healthy 26-year-old woman for a routine health visit. She mentions that she and her husband are thinking about starting a family soon. She has never been pregnant before. Which of the following interventions, if done prior to pregnancy, has been shown to have a clear beneficial outcome for this woman and her potential child?

a. Blood typing and antibody testing
b. Screening for HIV
c. Screening for *Chlamydia*
d. Screening for asymptomatic bacteriuria
e. Prescribing 0.4 to 0.8 mg of folic acid daily

17. You are discussing cancer screening with a patient. Her father was diagnosed with colorectal cancer at age 58. When should you recommend she begins colorectal cancer screening?

a. 40 years
b. 48 years
c. 50 years
d. 58 years
e. 60 years

18. You are discussing cancer screening with a female patient. She has no family history of breast cancer. At what age should she start getting routine mammograms?

a. 30 years
b. 35 years
c. 40 years
d. 45 years
e. 50 years

19. In a routine examination, a 33-year-old woman asks you about self breast examination as breast cancer screening method. Which of the following best represents current recommendations for breast self-examination (BSE)?

a. There is strong evidence that BSE is an appropriate screening modality.
b. There is no evidence that BSE is an appropriate screening modality.
c. There is insufficient evidence to recommend for or against BSE.
d. There is no evidence that BSE is an inappropriate screening modality.
e. There is strong evidence that BSE is an inappropriate screening modality.

20. A 52-year-old man comes to your office for a complete physical examination. He is interested in prostate cancer screening. Which of the following best represents current guidelines for prostate cancer screening?

a. There is insufficient evidence to recommend for or against prostate cancer screening.
b. Screening should consist of a digital rectal examination.
c. Screening should consist of a serum prostate specific antigen (PSA) test.
d. Screening should consist of both, a DRE and a serum PSA test.
e. Screening should include a CT scan of the prostate in high-risk individuals.

21. You are seeing a 40-year-old healthy man for a routine health examination. He is completely healthy, takes no medications, and has no abnormal physical examination findings. What are the current recommendations regarding obtaining a screening electrocardiogram (ECG) as part of his routine physical?

a. Recommendations strongly support obtaining a screening ECG
b. Recommendations weakly support obtaining a screening ECG
c. Recommendations do not support or oppose obtaining a screening ECG
d. Recommendations weakly oppose obtaining a screening ECG
e. Recommendations strongly oppose obtaining a screening ECG

22. During a routine appointment to discuss an upper respiratory infection, you find that your 18-year-old female patient has become sexually active for the first time. According to current guidelines, when should you begin cervical cancer screening on this patient?

a. At the current time.
b. At the age of 19.
c. At the age of 20.
d. At the age of 21.
e. Cervical cancer screening is not recommended.

23. You are seeing a 55-year-old patient for her annual physical examination. She has been married to her husband for 32 years and reports that both have been monogamous. She has never had an abnormal Pap smear. At what age is it appropriate to discontinue Pap screening on this patient?

a. 55 years.
b. 60 years.
c. 65 years.
d. 70 years.
e. Never discontinue screening.

24. You are caring for a healthy woman whose cousin was just diagnosed with unilateral breast cancer at age 33. Your patient has no other relatives with known histories of breast or ovarian cancer. Which of the following is true regarding the current recommendations for genetic screening for breast cancer mutations?

a. The patient should not be offered testing.
b. The patient should be tested only if she is of Ashkenazi Jewish descent.
c. The patient should be offered testing only if she is of Ashkenazi Jewish descent.
d. The patient should be tested regardless of her ethnicity.
e. The patient should be offered testing regardless of her ethnicity.

The Preoperative Evaluation

25. A 76-year-old male patient of yours is undergoing a left knee replacement for severe arthritis, and you are asked to perform his presurgical clearance. His past medical history is significant for episodic rate-controlled atrial fibrillation, a stroke at age 72 (from which he recovered fully), and uncontrolled hypertension. Last year, an echocardiogram showed he had severe aortic stenosis, but he has elected not to undergo surgical repair. He reports that he is sedentary, and is not able to walk up one flight of steps carrying his groceries without stopping to rest. His blood pressure upon evaluation is 168/92 mm Hg. Which of the described features are clinical predictors of increased perioperative cardiovascular risk for this surgery?

a. Advanced age
b. Rate-controlled atrial fibrillation
c. Uncontrolled hypertension
d. Severe aortic stenosis
e. Poor functional capacity

26. You are concerned about the cardiac risks of several of your patients undergoing surgical procedures, and are considering further cardiac testing in the preoperative period. Which of the following surgical procedures is considered to have a low surgery-specific risk, and generally does not require additional preoperative cardiac testing, if the patient does not have clinical predictors of increased cardiac risk?

a. Femoral-popliteal bypass
b. Breast surgery
c. Thyroidectomy
d. Knee replacement
e. Carotid endarterectomy

27. You are doing a preoperative history and physical examination on a 58-year-old woman who will be undergoing a cholecystectomy later in the month. She is obese, sedentary with type 2 diabetes, hyperlipidemia, and has a history of congestive heart failure in the past. She reports that she is unable to walk four blocks without stopping to rest. She denies chest pain with activity. Which of her historical features has been shown to have minimal negative impact on her postoperative outcome?

a. Obesity
b. Functional capacity
c. Type 2 diabetes
d. Hyperlipidemia
e. Congestive heart failure

28. You are doing a routine preoperative clearance for an otherwise healthy 60-year-old man undergoing a knee replacement. Which of the following laboratory tests should be ordered?

a. Hemoglobin
b. Electrolytes
c. Blood glucose
d. Serum creatinine
e. Urinalysis

29. A 50-year-old male patient is presenting for preoperative testing before undergoing arthroscopic knee surgery. Which of the following is true regarding ordering a preoperative ECG for this patient?

a. The patient should have a preoperative ECG done regardless of history or physical examination.
b. The patient should have a preoperative ECG done if he has a family history of hypertension.
c. The patient should have a preoperative ECG done if he has a family history of coronary artery disease.
d. The patient should have a preoperative ECG done if he is found to have elevated blood pressure during the preoperative evaluation.
e. The patient should have a preoperative ECG done if he has a history of tobacco use.

Travel Medicine

30. You are counseling one of your patients who is planning a trip overseas. He is concerned about becoming ill while traveling. Which of the following is the most common illness reported by international travelers?

a. Diarrhea
b. Upper respiratory infection
c. Parasitic infection
d. Malaria
e. Hepatitis

31. You are counseling a patient who is planning a trip with his wife to celebrate their 30th anniversary. They are going on an African safari, and wonder about health risks associated with international travel. What would you tell him is the most common cause of death among international travelers?

a. Infections
b. Accidents
c. Homicide
d. Heart disease
e. Vascular disease (ie, deep venous thrombosis and pulmonary embolus)

32. You are performing a physical examination on a student traveling to Mexico with her college Spanish class. She is concerned about traveler's diarrhea, and asks about antibiotic prophylaxis. Which of the following best represents the current guideline from the Centers for Disease Control (CDC) for prevention of traveler's diarrhea?

a. The CDC does not have an antibiotic guideline regarding antibiotic prophylaxis for traveler's diarrhea.
b. The traveler should take trimethoprim-sulfamethoxazole.
c. The traveler should take doxycycline.
d. The traveler should take ciprofloxacin.
e. The traveler should take metronidazole.

33. You are discussing vaccinations for a patient who is traveling internationally. Due to a significant fear of needles, he is unwilling to obtain any vaccination unless he feels there is significant risk of acquiring the condition. Which of the following vaccine preventable illness is most commonly acquired by travelers?

a. Yellow fever
b. Polio
c. Hepatitis A
d. Cholera
e. Typhus

34. You are discussing required vaccinations for an HIV infected traveler. Which of the following vaccines is recommended for immunodeficient patients?

a. Yellow fever vaccine
b. Inactivated polio vaccine
c. Cholera vaccine
d. Oral typhoid vaccine
e. MMR vaccine

Contraception

35. You are reevaluating a 32-year-old woman in your office. You started her on combination oral contraceptives (COCs) 3 months ago, and at each of three visits since then, her blood pressure has been elevated. Which of the following is the most appropriate next step?

a. Discontinue the oral contraceptive and recommend a barrier method.
b. Change to a pill with a higher estrogen component.
c. Change to a pill with a lower estrogen component.
d. Change to a pill with a lower progestin component.
e. Change to a progestin-only pill.

36. Which side effect of COCs is most frequently cited as the reason for discontinuing their use?

a. Nausea
b. Breast tenderness
c. Fluid retention
d. Headache
e. Irregular bleeding

37. You are counseling a 23-year-old woman who is interested in starting COC pills. Which of the following is true regarding risks associated with COC use?

a. Users of COC pills have an increased risk of ovarian cancer.
b. Users of COC pills have an increased risk of endometrial cancer.
c. Users of COC pills have an increased risk of venous thromboembolism.
d. Users of COC pills have an increased risk of hemorrhagic stroke.
e. Users of COC pills have an increased risk of diabetes mellitus.

√ **38.** A 29-year-old obese woman with type 2 diabetes mellitus is asking you about progestin-only pills as a method of contraception. Which of the following is true?

a. Progestin-only pills are contraindicated in women with diabetes.
b. Progestin-only pills would increase her risk of thromboembolic events.
c. Progestin-only pills are only Food and Drug Administration (FDA) approved for nursing women.
d. Progestin-only pills increase her risk for ectopic pregnancy.
e. Progestin-only pills should be taken every day of the month, without a hormone free period.

39. You are counseling a patient regarding contraception options. She is 36 years old, she smokes, weighs 145 lb, and has no medical illnesses. She is sexually active, but is not in a monogamous relationship. Which of the following is her best contraception option?

a. COC pills
b. An intravaginal ring system delivering estrogen and progestin
c. A transdermal contraceptive patch delivering estrogen and progestin
d. An injectable form of long-acting progestin
e. An intrauterine device (IUD)

40. A 28-year-old monogamous married woman comes to you for emergency contraception. She and her husband typically use condoms to prevent pregnancy, but when they had sex two evenings ago, the condom broke. She does not want to start a family at this time. Which of the following statements is true regarding the use of emergency contraception pills (ECPs)?

a. She is too late to use ECPs in this case.
b. ECPs are 90% to 100% effective when used correctly.
c. There are no medical contraindications to the use of ECPs, other than allergy or hypersensitivity to the pill components.
d. ECPs disrupt the pregnancy, if given within days of implantation.
e. Clinicians should perform a pregnancy test before prescribing ECPs.

Genetics and Pharmacogenomics

41. Consider the following pedigree:

Pedigree 1

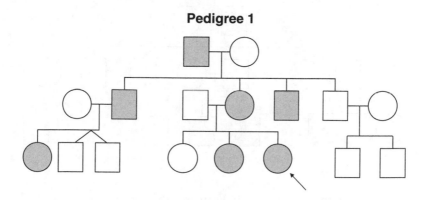

Assuming that the solid circles indicate that the persons are affected with the condition in question, which of the following is true regarding this condition?

a. It is autosomal dominant.
b. It is autosomal recessive.
c. It is X-linked recessive.
d. It is X-linked dominant.
e. It is unlikely to be a genetic disorder.

42. Consider the following pedigree:

Pedigree 2

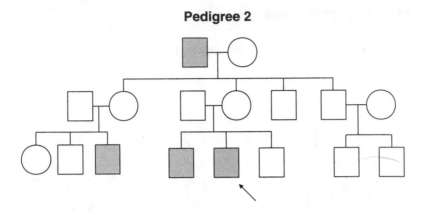

Assuming that the solid squares indicate that the persons are affected with the condition in question, which of the following is true regarding this condition?

a. It is autosomal dominant.
b. It is autosomal recessive.
c. It is X-linked recessive.
d. It is X-linked dominant.
e. It is unlikely to be a genetic disorder.

43. You are caring for a 45-year-old man with fatigue. Workup revealed hereditary hemochromatosis, an autosomal recessive disorder. Neither of his parents ever showed signs of the disease, though they were never tested while alive. Your patient has one sister. What is the chance that his sister is affected?

a. No chance
b. 10% chance
c. 25% chance
d. 50% chance
e. 100% chance

44. You are caring for a young family who just had a child with multiple malformations of unknown etiology. What type of testing would be best for identifying the diagnosis?

a. Cytogenetic analysis
b. Direct DNA testing
c. Biochemical testing
d. Linkage analysis
e. Protein-specific testing

Biostatistics

45. You note that in your practice, a large number of women with a family history of breast cancer in a first-degree relative develop breast cancer themselves. You evaluate a number of charts, and find that 5% of the women in your practice who have breast cancer have a family history, but only 2% of women without breast cancer have a family history. Given this information, what is the sensitivity of using family history as a predictor of breast cancer in your patient population?

a. 2%
b. 5%
c. 93%
d. 95%
e. 98%

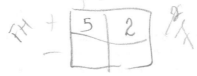

46. You are reading a population study that reports 90% of people with lung cancer are smokers. Thirty percent of the people without lung cancer are also smokers. Given this information, what is the specificity using smoking as a predictor of lung cancer?

a. 10%
b. 30%
c. 40%
d. 70%
e. 90%

47. You are determining whether or not to use a rapid streptococcal antigen test to screen for streptococcal pharyngitis. You find that 2% of people with strep throat actually test negative using this test. Which of the following statements best describes this situation?

a. The sensitivity of the test is 2%.
b. The specificity of the test is 98%.
c. The test has a 2% false-negative rate.
d. The test has a 2% false-positive rate.
e. The test has a positive predictive value of 98%.

48. You are reading a medical journal and come across an article about diabetes. The study followed 10,000 patients over 3 years. At the start of the study, 2000 people had diabetes. At the end of the study, 1000 additional people developed diabetes. What was the incidence of diabetes during the study?

a. 10%
b. 12.5%
c. 20%
d. 30%
e. 50%

49. You are reading a study that compares cholesterol levels in children whose fathers died from a myocardial infarction with cholesterol levels in children whose fathers died from other causes. The p value obtained in the test was <0.001. What does this value indicate?

a. There was no difference in cholesterol levels between the two groups.
b. The difference in the cholesterol levels was less than 0.1%.
c. There is a less than 0.1% probability that the results obtained in this study were incorrect.
d. There is a less than 0.1% probability that the results obtained in this study occurred because of a sampling error.
e. If the null hypothesis is true, there is a less than 0.1% probability of obtaining a test statistic equal to or more extreme than the one obtained.

50. You are considering using a new influenza screening test. You find a study that evaluated 1000 patients with this new test. Of these 1000 patients, 400 had the disease. Three hundred of those had positive tests, and 100 of those had a negative test. Of the 600 that did not have the disease, 200 had positive tests, and 400 had negative tests. What is the positive predictive value of this test?

a. 50%
b. 60%
c. 66%
d. 75%
e. 80%

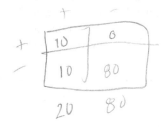

51. You find that many of your patients that have gone to the emergency department with chest pain have a negative set of initial cardiac enzymes. Most of those with a negative set of initial enzymes did not have a heart attack. You decide to evaluate 100 of your patients who have gone to the emergency department with chest pain to find out if an initial set of negative enzymes by itself is a good predictor of those that are not having a myocardial infarction (MI). Of those 100 patients, 20 of them had acute MIs. Of those 20, 10 had a positive set of enzymes initially. Of the 80 that did not have an acute MI, none of them had a positive set of initial enzymes. Given this information, what is the negative predictive value of the initial set of cardiac enzymes in your patient population?

a. 20%
b. 22%
c. 50%
d. 89%
e. 100%

Preventive Medicine

Answers

1. The answer is c. (*Lee, 2006.*) Without intervention, up to 90% of children born of mothers who are positive for hepatitis B surface antigen and hepatitis B antigen will have chronic hepatitis B by 6 months of age. Studies have shown that compared to no intervention, treating the infant with hepatitis B immune globulin within 12 hours of birth, and vaccination, reduces that infection rate by more than 50%. Therefore, all mothers should be screened for hepatitis B surface antigen, and if positive, the babies should be treated as described in this question. If the hepatitis status of the mother is unknown, the child should get the vaccine, and the mother should be tested. If found to be positive, the baby should receive immune globulin within 7 days.

2. The answer is a. (*Yeh.*) Prior to the introduction of an effective vaccine, Hib was the most common cause of bacterial meningitis and a frequent cause of other bacteremic infections, particularly in childhood. The use of the vaccine has led to a dramatic decrease of invasive Hib disease. In fact, in countries where the vaccine is widely used, invasive Hib has been virtually eliminated. The vaccine does not reduce the rate of otitis media, as most cases are due to nontypeable *H influenzae*. Adverse reactions to the vaccine are very rare. In fact, no serious reactions have been linked to the vaccine, and systemic reactions like fever and irritability are infrequent. The vaccine should not be administered before 6 weeks of age, as immune tolerance to the antigen may be induced. The vaccine may be given with other vaccines.

3. The answer is b. (*ACIP, 2007.*) Varicella-zoster infection is more severe in neonates and adults. After one dose of vaccine, breakthrough cases are common, and therefore two doses are recommended. While many people who do not remember having chicken pox have serologic evidence of immunity, testing is not necessary, as the vaccine is well-tolerated in those already immune. No special precautions are necessary for households with immunocompromised persons, unless the person vaccinated develops a rash. Zoster is more common among those with natural infection as opposed to those who were immunized.

4. The answer is a. *(Rakel, pp 182-193.)* Hepatitis B vaccination is recommended for nonimmune people who are high-risk. These include men who have sex with men, people with multiple sexual partners, sex industry workers, intravenous drug users, prison inmates, people on hemodialysis, people living in households with hepatitis B virus carriers, health care workers, and people from endemic areas. In this question, having a positive surface antibody means that the patient is immune. If the patient were to be negative, the immunization schedule would be one injection at time 0, one between 1 to 2 months after that, and a third injection between 4 to 6 months after the second.

5. The answer is c. *(Rakel, pp 182-193.)* Hepatitis A vaccination is indicated for men who have sex with men or users of illegal drugs. The patient is not at high risk for varicella, and therefore vaccination is not indicated. Meningitis vaccination is indicated for those with functional asplenia or travelers to endemic areas. College students can be counseled about the vaccination, especially if they are living in a dormitory. Pneumococcal vaccination is only indicated for those with chronic diseases, functional asplenia or residents of long-term care facilities. An MMR booster is not indicated.

6. The answer is d. *(Rakel, pp 182-193.)* Congenital rubella syndrome is devastating, and rubella immunity is important for women considering pregnancy. If a woman is found to be rubella nonimmune, vaccination should not occur if she is pregnant or planning pregnancy in the next 4 weeks. If she is currently pregnant and nonimmune, she should be vaccinated as early in the postpartum period as possible.

7. The answer is e. *(McPhee, pp 1-18.)* Increasing reports of pertussis among US adults has stimulated vaccine development for older persons. A tetanus-diphtheria 5-component acellular pertussis vaccine (Tdap) is available, and recommended for adults age 19 to 64 to replace the next booster dose of tetanus.

8. The answer is c. *(Rakel, pp 182-193.)* Influenza vaccination is recommended annually for children ages 6 months and older with certain risk factors (asthma, cardiac disease, sickle-cell disease, HIV, and diabetes among others). It can be administered to all others wishing to obtain immunity as well. In addition, children between 6 to 24 months should be offered the vaccine, as they are at substantial risk for hospitalization if infected. In this case, since the mother wishes all her children be vaccinated, only the 4-month-old should be excluded because of age.

9. The answer is e. *(ACIP, 2008.)* The CDC Advisory Committee on Immunization Practices (ACIP) updated its recommendation for the use of the 7-valent pneumococcal vaccination (PCV7) in children under 5 years of age that have not been vaccinated. This recommendation states that all healthy children, age 24 to 59 months that have not completed their primary immunization for PCV7 be given one dose of PCV7. If the child had received less than three doses of the PCV7 during his/her primary immunization series, two doses should be given at least 8 weeks apart. The usual schedule for the series is one vaccination at 2, 4, 6, and 12 to 15 months.

10. The answer is d. *(ACIP, 2007a.)* The HPV vaccination is recommended for all adult women under the age of 26 who have not completed the vaccine series. History of genital warts or an abnormal Pap test are not, by themselves, evidence of prior infection with all HPV subtypes, and are not reasons to avoid vaccination. Persons who are sexually active but not in monogamous relationships are at risk for infection, and should therefore be immunized if they meet criteria.

11. The answer is c. *(ACIP, 2007b.)* The quadrivalent HPV vaccination has been shown to be highly immunogenic, safe, and well-tolerated in females age 9 to 26, in studies. To be most effective, the vaccine should be given before a female becomes sexually active. It can be administered when a patient has an abnormal Pap test or when a woman is breast-feeding. It can also be given when a patient is immunocompromised because of a disease or medication. It is not recommended for use during pregnancy.

12. The answer is d. *(ACIP, 2007a.)* Of the vaccines listed, only the pneumococcal polysaccharide vaccine is indicated for people who have chronic pulmonary disease. She should receive a one-time administration, since she is over the age of 65. Had she received her initial shot before the age of 65, she would require a one-time "booster" shot, 5 years after the initial one. People born before 1957 do not need to be vaccinated with an MMR, as they are considered immune. People born before 1980 are considered immune to varicella. The Tdap vaccine is only indicated for those under the age of 65, and intranasal influenza should only be used in healthy adults under the age of 50.

13. The answer is e. (*ACIP, 2007a.*) The herpes zoster vaccination is currently recommended for adults 60 years of age or older regardless of whether or not they report a prior episode of herpes zoster. The vaccination is not approved for persons under the age of 60, though trials are currently underway to assess safety and efficacy in younger age groups.

14. The answer is d. (*American Academy of Family Physicians, 2008.*) Determining which screening tests are appropriate for a patient is difficult, and requires individual judgment based on the clinical situation. The American Academy of Family Physicians has developed clinical preventive services charts based on age alone in low-risk adults, and rank the screen as "strongly recommend," "recommend," and "healthy behavior." Strongly recommended screens are supported by good quality evidence and demonstrate substantial net benefit for the patient. It is strongly recommended that men are screened for lipid disorders at age 35, even in the absence of other risk factors. Screening would occur earlier in the presence of diabetes, a family history of heart disease by age 50, or with other risk factors.

15. The answer is a. (*American Academy of Family Physicians, 2008.*) The US Preventive Services Task Force has found that CT scanning, chest x-ray, and sputum cytology can detect lung cancer at an earlier stage than no screening at all, but also found no evidence that any screening strategy actually improves mortality. Therefore, no screening is recommended for this patient.

16. The answer is e. (*American Academy of Family Physicians, 2008.*) Of the interventions listed above, only prescribing folic acid has been shown to be beneficial prior to pregnancy. It will decrease the chance of neural tube defects in the baby. The other interventions should be done early in the pregnancy to ensure good pregnancy outcome.

17. The answer is b. (*American Academy of Family Physicians, 2008.*) In general, colorectal cancer screening should begin at age 50. In cases where there is a family history of colorectal cancer, the screen should begin 10 years before the cancer was diagnosed in the family, or at age 50, whichever is sooner.

18. The answer is c. (*American Academy of Family Physicians, 2008.*) Mammograms (with or without clinical breast examinations) have clearly been shown to reduce mortality associated with breast cancer. Guidelines vary, but the US Preventive Services Task Force recommends routine mammography every 1 to 2 years beginning at age 40.

19. The answer is c. (*American Academy of Family Physicians, 2008.*) The American Academy of Family Physicians has concluded that there is insufficient evidence to recommend for or against using BSE as a screening modality. Evidence is poor that BSE reduces mortality, and there is fairly strong evidence that BSE is associated with an increased risk for false-positive results and biopsies. Due to limitations in published and ongoing studies, the balance between benefits and harm is not known.

20. The answer is a. (*American Academy of Family Physicians, 2008.*) There is evidence supporting DRE and PSA testing as a prostate cancer screen, but concerns exist regarding false-positive tests and any actual reduction in mortality that is gained from doing the tests. Therefore, the American Academy of Family Physicians feels the evidence is insufficient to recommend for or against routine prostate cancer screening. In patients who are interested in screening, physicians should discuss the potential benefits and harms with the patients before making a decision to test.

21. The answer is e. (*American Academy of Family Physicians, 2008.*) The American Academy of Family Physicians recommends against the routine use of the ECG as part of periodic health or preparticipation examinations in asymptomatic adults. There is no evidence that the use of ECG screening improves mortality or identification of asymptomatic disease.

22. The answer is d. (*American Academy of Family Physicians, 2008.*) There is a strong recommendation from the American Academy of Family Physicians for cervical cancer screening at least every 3 years for women who have ever had sex and have a cervix. However, the optimal age at which to begin screening is unknown. Some recommend that screening should start at the onset of sexual activity or at age 18, whichever comes first. However, evidence, coupled with the natural history of HPV infection, indicates that screening can safely be delayed until 3 years after the onset of sexual activity or age 21, whichever comes first.

23. The answer is a. (*American Academy of Family Physicians, 2008.*) Guidelines for low-risk women indicate that Pap testing should be conducted at least every 3 years in women who have ever had sex and still have a cervix. The guidelines regarding when to discontinue testing are not as clear. However, the yield of the Pap test is low in women who have been previously screened at age 65. The American Cancer Society recommends discontinuing screening at age 70, but also notes that a woman who has had three or more documented normal, technically satisfactory Pap tests, and has had no abnormal Pap tests in the last 10 years can safely stop screening.

24. The answer is a. *(Isaacs.)* Two major susceptibility genes for breast cancer, *BRCA 1* and *BRCA 2* have been identified, and testing for these mutations is commercially available. However, testing is very expensive, and the interpretation of results is sometimes difficult. The prevalence of *BRCA* mutations is highest among women of Ashkenazi Jewish descent, and approximately 2% of those women carry a deleterious mutation. Current recommendations for genetic screening in women without a personal history of breast cancer are variable, however, the US Preventive Services Task Force guidelines state that a woman should be tested if she has:

- Two first-degree relatives with breast cancer, one of whom was diagnosed under the age of 50.
- A combination of three or more first- or second-degree relatives with breast cancer regardless of the age at diagnosis.
- A combination of breast and ovarian cancer among first- and second-degree relatives.
- A first-degree relative with bilateral breast cancer.
- A combination of two or more first- or second-degree relatives with ovarian cancer, regardless of age at diagnosis.
- A first- or second-degree relative with both breast and ovarian cancer at any age.
- A male relative with breast cancer.

Ashkenazi Jewish women should be offered testing if any first-degree relative (or two second-degree relatives on the same side of the family) are diagnosed with breast or ovarian cancer.

25. The answer is d. *(Shammash.)* Family physicians are often asked to perform preoperative evaluations for their patients. The purpose of these evaluations is to identify risks for poor outcomes that may not be immediately apparent to the surgeon. In 2002, the American College of Cardiology and the American Heart Association summarized clinical predictors for increased perioperative cardiovascular risk. They found that advanced age, a rhythm other than sinus rhythm (atrial fibrillation), uncontrolled hypertension, and low functional capacity were not proven to independently increase perioperative cardiovascular risk in low- or intermediate-risk surgeries.

However, severe heart valve disease was a major predictor of perioperative risk. Other major predictors are acute MI (within 7 days), recent MI (between 8 to 30 days), unstable or severe angina, decompensated heart failure, high grade A/V block, symptomatic arrhythmias with underlying heart disease, and supraventricular arrhythmias with a poorly controlled ventricular rate.

26. The answer is b. (*Shammash.*) When evaluating a patient's risk for undergoing a surgical procedure, the family physician must look at the patient-specific clinical variables, the patient's exercise capacity, and the risk of the surgical procedure being performed. High-risk surgical procedures are those with a risk of cardiac death greater than 5%, and include emergent operations, aortic or other major vascular surgeries, peripheral artery surgery, or prolonged surgeries with large anticipated fluid shifts. Intermediate-risk procedures have a risk of cardiac death between 1% to 5% and include carotid endarterectomies, head and neck surgeries, intrathoracic and intraperitoneal surgeries, orthopedic surgeries, and prostate surgeries. Low-risk procedures have a risk of cardiac death less than 1% and generally do not require additional cardiac preoperative testing. They include endoscopic procedures, superficial procedures, cataract surgeries, and breast surgery.

27. The answer is a. (*Smetana.*) Surprisingly, obesity is not a risk factor for adverse postoperative outcomes. Type 2 diabetes, hyperlipidemia, and congestive heart failure may all require additional preoperative testing. Poor functional capacity is defined as being unable to walk four blocks or up two flights of steps. Persons with poor functional capacity have more than twice as many adverse outcomes than their counterparts with better functional capacity.

28. The answer is d. (*Smetana.*) Random preoperative laboratory testing can increase costs, have little benefit, and have a high rate of false-positive tests. Therefore, selective use of laboratory tests is a more prudent approach. In general, guidelines suggest a hemoglobin or hematocrit for surgery with expected major blood loss and electrolytes only if the patient has a history that increases the likelihood of an abnormality (diuretic use). Routine blood glucose and urinalysis measurements are not recommended. Serum creatinine should be tested if the surgery is major, hypotension is expected, nephrotoxic drugs will be used or the patient is above 50.

29. The answer is a. (*Smetana.*) Most experts agree that a preoperative ECG should be performed routinely in:

- Men older than 45 years.
- Women older than 55 years.
- Patients with a history of known cardiac disease.
- Patients with a clinical history suggesting cardiac disease.
- Patients at risk for electrolyte abnormalities, such as those using diuretics.
- Patients with systemic disease associated with unrecognized cardiac disease, such as hypertension or diabetes.
- Patients undergoing major surgical procedures.

In the case above, the patient's age indicated he would have an ECG regardless of the other factors identified in the history or physical.

30. The answer is a. (*Rakel, pp 193-204.*) Approximately 50 million people travel abroad each year. Of these, almost 50% will become ill while traveling. Traveler's diarrhea is the most common illness, followed by upper respiratory infection (URI), viral syndromes, skin conditions, parasitic infections, malaria, hepatitis, and other more rare infections.

31. The answer is d. (*Rakel, pp 193-204.*) Heart disease is the most common cause of death while traveling, likely because it is such a common cause of death in general. The second most common cause of death is accidents. People traveling engage in risky behavior that they otherwise might not indulge in. Dangerous recreation activities, increased drinking, driving in foreign countries all contribute to causing accidents. Discussing accident prevention is therefore the key when counseling patients planning to travel abroad.

32. The answer is a. (*Rakel, pp 193-204.*) The CDC does not recommend antibiotic chemoprophylaxis for traveler's diarrhea because of the development of resistant organisms. Most times, the condition is self-limited. The CDC does recommend using common sense regarding food and water, eating nothing unless it is boiled, peeled, or cooked.

33. The answer is c. (*Rakel, pp 193-204.*) Hepatitis A is the most common vaccine preventable illness acquired by travelers. Yellow fever is the only legally required immunization (and then, only for some countries). A single inactivated polio vaccine (IPV) booster is recommended for adult travelers who have had primary polio immunization, but who will be traveling to an area where polio is endemic. Cholera and typhus are generally not required immunizations for travelers.

34. The answer is b. *(Weller.)* Vaccines that contain live, attenuated viruses (yellow fever, oral polio, oral typhoid, and MMR vaccines) should not be given to immunocompromised patients. Inactivated polio is safe, as is the parenteral typhoid vaccine. Cholera immunization is no longer recommended for travelers.

35. The answer is a. *(South-Paul, pp 173-181.)* In some patients COCs cause a small increase in blood pressure. This risk increases with age. Both estrogen and progestin are known to cause blood pressure elevations, so changing formulations of COC or using progestin-only pills may not lead to problem resolution. Once COCs are discontinued, blood pressure usually returns to normal within 3 months.

36. The answer is e. *(South-Paul, pp 173-181.)* Side effects of COCs include androgenic effects (hair growth, male pattern baldness, nausea.) and estrogenic effects (nausea, breast tenderness, and fluid retention). Weight gain is thought to be a common side effect, but multiple studies have failed to show it to be a statistically significant side effect. The side effect most frequently cited as the reason for stopping use of COCs is irregular bleeding. It is common in the first 3 months of use, and generally diminishes over time.

37. The answer is c. *(South-Paul, pp 173-181.)* The use of COC pills is associated with a threefold risk of venous thromboembolism. COCs have a protective effect against ovarian cancer and endometrial cancer. The risk of hemorrhagic stroke is not increased by the use of COCs, and they have not been shown in studies to impact carbohydrate metabolism in a statistically significant way.

38. The answer is e. *(South-Paul, pp 173-181.)* Progestin-only pills prevent conception through suppression of ovulation, thickening of cervical mucus, alteration of the endometrium, and inhibition of tubal transport. The effectiveness of this method is dependent on consistency of use. In fact, if a pill is taken even 3 hours late, an alternative form of contraception should be used for 48 hours. There is no hormone-free period with these pills, and they should be taken every day. The pills do not carry an increased risk for thromboembolism, and the World Health Organization has reported this form of contraception to be safe for women with a history of venous thrombosis, pulmonary embolism, diabetes, obesity, or hypertension. Nursing women can use this pill, but there is FDA approval for use in others as well. In general, progestin-only pills protect against ectopic pregnancy by lowering the chance of conception. However, if progestin-only pill users get pregnant, the chance of ectopic pregnancy is 6% to 10%, higher than the rate found in women not using contraception. Therefore, users should be aware of the symptoms for ectopic pregnancy.

39. The answer is d. (*South-Paul, pp 173-181.*) Oral contraceptive pills containing estrogen and progestin components are contraindicated in smokers over the age of 35, due to an increased risk of thromboembolic events. An intravaginal ring or transdermal patch that releases estrogen and progestin are also contraindicated in smokers over the age of 35 for the same reason. IUDs should not be used in women with more than one sexual partner, or in people whose partner has more than one partner. IUDs should not be used in people at high risk for developing a sexually transmitted infection, as women with an IUD are more likely to develop pelvic inflammatory disease after a sexually transmitted infection as compared with those using hormonal methods. An injectable long acting progestin would therefore be the best choice in this woman.

40. The answer is c. (*South-Paul, pp 173-181.*) Emergency contraception is appropriate when no contraception was used (including cases of sexual assault), or when there is contraceptive failure. They should be used within 72 hours of intercourse, well before implantation (implantation occurs 5-7 days after intercourse). ECPs involve limited hormonal exposure, and therefore have not been shown to increase the risk of venous thromboembolism, stroke, or MI. In fact, there are no medical contraindications to the use of emergency contraception pills. They do not disrupt an already implanted pregnancy and do not cause birth defects. Progestin ECPs prevent 85% of expected pregnancies when used correctly, and combined ECPs prevent 75% of expected pregnancies. They are not 100% effective in pregnancy prevention. There is no need to perform a pregnancy test when prescribing.

41. The answer is a. (*South-Paul, pp 533-542.*) The pedigree shown is for an autosomal dominant condition. As the pedigree shows, males and females in the family are equally affected, and parents are transmitting the gene to their offspring (vertical inheritance). If this were an autosomal recessive trait, horizontal inheritance would be more present, with multiple children being affected from unaffected parents. X-linked recessive traits affect more males than females, and X-linked dominant traits affect more females than males.

42. The answer is c. (*South-Paul, pp 533-542.*) The pedigree shown is for an X-linked recessive condition. As the pedigree shows, the condition affects more males than females, and inheritance is through the maternal side of the family (diagonal inheritance). Female carriers have a 50% risk for each daughter to be a carrier and a 50% risk for each son to be affected. All daughters of an affected male are carriers, and none of his sons are affected. If this were an autosomal dominant condition, males and females would be equally affected, and parents would transmit the gene to their offspring. If this were an autosomal recessive trait, horizontal inheritance would be present, with multiple children being affected from unaffected parents. If it were X-linked dominant, more females would be affected than males.

43. The answer is c. (*South-Paul, pp 533-542.*) In the case of an autosomal recessive trait, if unaffected parents have an affected child, there is a 25% risk that each offspring from those parents will be affected. Both parents must be carriers of the trait, which means that each child born to them has a 25% risk of not carrying the gene, a 50% risk of being a carrier, and a 25% risk of having the disease.

44. The answer is a. (*South-Paul, pp 533-542.*) Cytogenetic analysis is a microscopic study of the chromosomes and is used to identify abnormalities in chromosome number, size, or structure. It is commonly ordered when patients are suspected of having a recognizable chromosomal syndrome (trisomy 21) and in newborns with multiple malformations of unknown etiology or with ambiguous genitalia. Direct DNA testing is indicated for patients affected or predisposed to a condition for which the gene change that causes the condition has been identified (cystic fibrosis). Biochemical tests identify or quantify metabolites or enzymes to measure activity, and are commonly used to diagnose and monitor disorders of metabolism. Linkage analyses identify genetic sequences that are physically in close proximity to a disease gene of interest.

45. The answer is b. *(Rosner, pp 43-67.)* Sensitivity is thought of as the probability that a symptom is present given that the person has the disease. In the above example, the "symptom" in question is a family history of breast cancer. Of women that have breast cancer, 5% have a family history; therefore the sensitivity of using family history as a predictor of breast cancer is 5%.

46. The answer is d. *(Rosner, pp 43-67.)* Specificity can be thought of as the probability that the symptom is *not* present given that a person does not have a disease. In the above example, the "symptom" is smoking. Of people who do not have lung cancer, 30% of them are smokers, indicating that 70% of them are not smokers. Of the people who do not have lung cancer, 70% of them do not smoke.

47. The answer is c. *(Rosner, pp 43-67.)* A false-negative is defined as a person who tests negative, but who is actually positive. In the above example, 2% of the positive people test negative. Therefore, the false-negative rate is 2% in this case. Sensitivity is defined as the probability that the test would be positive, given that the person has strep throat. The specificity is the probability that the test would be negative if the person does *not* have strep. The false-positive rate is defined as the percent of people who test positive, but are actually negative. The positive predictive value is the probability that a person has an illness, given that the test is positive.

48. The answer is b. *(Rosner, pp 43-67.)* The incidence of a disease is the probability that a person with no prior disease will develop a new case of the disease over a specific time period. In this case, 1000 people developed diabetes. In the study, only 8000 people began with no prior disease. Therefore, the incidence is 1000/8000 or 12.5%. The prevalence is the probability of having a disease at a specific point in time, and is obtained by dividing the number of people with the disease by the number of people in the study.

49. The answer is e. *(Rosner, pp 296-337.)* The *p* value for any hypothesis test is the level at which we would be indifferent between accepting or rejecting the null hypothesis given the sample data at hand. It can also be thought of as the probability of obtaining a test statistic as extreme or more extreme than the actual test statistic obtained, given that the null hypothesis is true. It does not reflect the absolute difference in the data between groups, and does not reflect the *correctness* of the data in the sample.

50. The answer is b. (*Mahutte.*) The positive predictive value refers to the probability that a positive test correctly identifies an individual who actually has the disease. Using a 4 × 4 chart:

	Disease present	Disease absent	Total
Test positive	A = 300	B = 200	500
Test negative	C = 100	D = 400	500
Total	400	600	**1000**
Positive predictive value = A/(A+B), or 300/500 = 60%			

51. The answer is d. (*Mahutte.*) The negative predictive value is the probability that a negative test correctly identifies an individual who does not have the disease. Using a 4 × 4 chart:

	Disease present	Disease absent	Total
Test positive	A = 10	B = 0	10
Test negative	C = 10	D = 80	90
Total	20	80	**100**
Negative predictive value = D/(C+D), or 80/90 = 89%			

Doctor-Patient Issues

Questions

Communication

52. You are performing a medical interview with a patient and having some difficulty obtaining accurate information regarding the events that brought him into the office. Which of the following physician communication tactics leads to the collection of the most accurate information?

a. Controlling the interview with more directive questions.
b. Using medical terms that the physician feels the patient can understand.
c. Redirecting the patient if he/she strays from the relevant points.
d. Involving the patient in his/her treatment plan.
e. Using open-ended questions.

53. You were involved in a minor motor vehicle accident on the way to work. As a result, you saw your first patient of the morning more than 1 hour after the scheduled appointment time. When you walk in, he appears extremely angry. Which of the following alternatives is the most patient-centered way to approach this situation?

a. Explain what happened so that he will understand why you are late.
b. Acknowledge his anger with a statement like, "You seem very angry."
c. Apologize for the delay and efficiently take care of his problem.
d. Explore the reasons for his anger if he brings it up.
e. Help the patient understand that his anger should be directed at his illness, not at you.

54. You are having trouble caring for a 58-year-old woman with uncontrolled diabetes. Her measures of glucose control are always significantly higher than you'd like to see, and you feel that she may not be taking her medications as directed. Which of the following is the most effective way to measure her adherence to the prescribed medical regimen?

a. Ask her if she is taking her medications.
b. Look for a reduction in her blood glucose measurements in subsequent visits.
c. Have her bring in her medications so that you may perform pill counts.
d. Measure serum blood levels of her medications.
e. Ask her specific questions about her medication names, dosages, and administration times.

55. You are seeing a 65-year-old woman who has smoked for 50 years. You want her to quit, and are considering different communication tactics to use in the discussion. Which of the following is likely to be the most powerful motivator?

a. Point out the positive results that can be expected if she complies with your advice. "By quitting, you'll significantly reduce your chances of developing lung cancer."
b. Point out the consequences of not following your advice. "If you don't quit, you might develop lung cancer."
c. Empathize. "I'll bet that quitting is extremely difficult."
d. Provide data. "Evidence shows that 1 in 20 patients who try can quit smoking cold turkey."
e. Ask about their experience with the illness that she is at risk for. "Do you know anyone who has ever suffered with emphysema?"

56. A 23-year-old man is following up to discuss the results of laboratory tests you did at his complete physical examination 1 week ago. His human immunodeficiency virus (HIV) screen was positive, and you need to tell him this news. Which of the following is the most appropriate approach?

a. Begin the session by inquiring about his understanding of HIV.
b. Help him prepare for the information by using a statement like, "I'm afraid I have some bad news for you."
c. Ensure you schedule enough time to discuss treatment goals and options.
d. Make sure he brings a support person into the room before you disclose the test results.
e. Offer hope by saying, "I'm sure there will be a cure for this disease soon."

✓**57.** Regarding patient education and counseling, which of the following statements is true?

a. Patients usually understand and remember most information from their physician.
b. Patients commonly believe that physicians give them too much information.
c. Patients are more likely to make behavior changes if they are given several options for change from which to choose.
d. Physician eye contact does not improve patient recall.
e. Patients feel patronized when physicians repeat information.

Cultural Competency and Health Disparities

58. You are treating a 61-year-old Chinese immigrant. You diagnose type 2 diabetes, but the patient is reluctant to make the dietary changes necessary to help treat the condition, as much of her high glycemic index diet is culturally based. Which of the following is the most culturally appropriate approach?

a. Ask to involve her Americanized children in future communication to help encourage the changes.
b. Since her culture believes that health is a balance between yin and yang, tell her that the dietary changes you suggest will restore this balance.
c. Organize an appointment with the patient and a diabetes educator who can better take the time and explain the etiology and dietary regimen necessary for diabetes.
d. Inquire as to the patient's concept of the etiology of diabetes and any treatments she would like to try.
e. Use a Chinese interpreter to ensure your message is being heard appropriately.

✓**59.** You are caring for a patient originally from Mexico, and are communicating with the help of a Spanish-speaking interpreter. Which of the following statements is true regarding the effective use of an interpreter?

a. Ask the interpreter to explain your statements, when necessary.
b. Arrange seats in a triad, and speak slowly, facing the interpreter.
c. Act as if the interpreter is not present, speaking to the patient normally.
d. Use as many nonverbal gestures as possible.
e. If you get an unexpected response, repeat the same question over again.

60. You are interacting with a patient who has emigrated from Russia. The patient is not complying with the treatment plan you outlined for his hyperlipidemia. Which of the following is the most effective way to improve this situation?

a. Speak with Russian colleagues to better understand the Russian culture.
b. Refer the patient to a physician from the same cultural background as the patient.
c. Study the Russian culture as it relates to illness and healing, and offer alternatives for treatment consistent with the cultural norms.
d. Listen to the patient's perspective, express your treatment plan, and focus on similarities and differences.
e. Examine the cultures beliefs of Russians and use these beliefs to convince the patient to comply with treatment.

61. You are working at a medical office whose population includes a large proportion of Native American patients. Which of the following health issues has a higher prevalence in this population than in other American population groups?

a. Hypertension
b. Coronary artery disease
c. Obesity
d. Asthma
e. Tuberculosis

62. You are working in an office that provides care to a large population of homeless patients. Which is true about medical illnesses in homeless children as compared with other groups of children?

a. Homeless children are more likely to develop type 2 diabetes.
b. Homeless children experience a higher number of ear infections.
c. Homeless children are more likely to have chronic illness.
d. Homeless children are more likely to have depression.
e. Homeless children are more likely to have attention deficit disorders.

63. You are working in an office that serves a large uninsured population. Which of the following is true regarding this population as compared to the privately insured population?

a. This population has fewer chronic health conditions.
b. This population has a lower mortality rate.
c. This population has a better general health status.
d. This population has a better mental health status.
e. This population has a higher rate of chronic disease among children.

64. You are evaluating health disparities in your community and using mortality rates as a measure of overall health. Which of the following population subgroups in the United States has the lowest mortality rate at each age of the lifespan?

a. African Americans
b. Hispanic Americans
c. Native Americans
d. Asian Americans
e. Non-Hispanic whites

65. You are evaluating a Hispanic patient with multiple somatic complaints and suspect a mental health disorder. Which of the following is true regarding mental health disparities in the United States today?

a. Mental health disorders are diagnosed less frequently in minority populations than in non-Hispanic white patients.
b. It is uncommon for minority groups to express mental health disorders via somatization.
c. Minority patients are more likely to be misdiagnosed than nonminority counterparts.
d. Minorities who maintain cultural practices and resist involvement in the dominant culture have better mental health.
e. Culture is less of a factor in mental health than in other organic syndromes or illnesses.

Ethics and Professionalism

66. You are taking care of a 62-year-old woman with a urinary tract infection. You prescribe trimethoprim-sulfamethoxazole (Bactrim) for her infection, but forget to ask about her allergies. The next day, she returns with significant hives, asking if Bactrim contains "sulfa," something she is allergic to. Which of the following fundamental principles of medical professionalism has been violated?

a. The principle of primacy of patient welfare
b. The principle of patient autonomy
c. The principle of social justice
d. The principle of professional competence
e. The principle of honesty with patients

67. You are working with a physician who is treating a patient for hypertension. The patient has a documented allergy to angiotensin-converting enzyme inhibitors, and you note that the physician is prescribing them. You assume that the physician knows best, and do not let the physician know of the potential mistake. What professional responsibility have you violated?

a. Commitment to honesty with patients
b. Commitment to professional competence
c. Commitment to maintaining appropriate patient relationships
d. Commitment to improving quality of care
e. Commitment to maintaining trust

68. You are working as a student in the emergency room. After a cardiac arrest and a prolonged attempt at resuscitation, a patient dies. The attending physician asks if you would like to gain experience by practicing intubations on the patient who has died. You feel that this relates to one of your professional responsibilities, to maintain clinical competence, and consider the offer. Which fundamental principle of professionalism and ethics would be violated if you do this?

a. The principle of patient welfare
b. The principle of patient autonomy
c. The principle of social justice
d. The principle of honesty with patients
e. The principle of maintaining trust

69. In the elevator, your senior resident says, "Before I forget, make sure you send Mr. Davis home on his usual HIV medications." You know that there are new medications that he could take, that might give him a better antiviral response. There are other health care providers in the elevator. What professional responsibility has your senior resident violated?

a. Commitment to maintaining trust
b. Commitment to improving quality of care
c. Commitment to professional competence
d. Commitment to scientific knowledge
e. Commitment to patient confidentiality

70. One of your patients is 6 months pregnant, and is found to have a medical condition that, if left untreated, will be life-threatening to both her and the fetus. She believes that God will take care of her and the baby, and she refuses medical intervention offered to her. Which of the following best describes the principle of patient autonomy in this case?

a. She has no right to refuse the intervention, based on the fact that her decision is lethal to both her and her unborn infant.
b. She has no right to refuse the intervention, based on the fact that her decision is lethal to her infant.
c. She has the right to refuse the intervention regardless of the condition.
d. She has the right to refuse the intervention, only if the father of her baby agrees.
e. She has the right to refuse the intervention if she is found competent to make the decision.

71. You are caring for a 55-year-old man who recently has complained of chest pain. His electrocardiogram is abnormal, and you feel he should have a cardiac catheterization. After explaining the risks and benefits to him, he refuses the intervention. Which of the following responses best demonstrates the tenets of professionalism in this case?

a. Respect the patient's choice and continue to explore his reasons for refusing treatment.
b. Explain to him that you think he is making a bad decision, and try to convince him to change his mind.
c. Consult the ethics committee of the hospital.
d. Consult a psychiatrist to determine the patient's competency.
e. Discharge the patient from your practice because of the poor doctor-patient relationship you have with him.

72. You are caring for a 38-year-old man with metastatic cancer. He thoroughly understands his condition, and realizes that he has only a few months to live. He asks that you do not tell his wife about his prognosis, as "she won't be able to take it." The patient's wife sees you in the hallway and says, "tell me the truth . . . how is his condition?" Which of the following responses best reflects an ethically sound course of action?

a. Tell her the truth about the situation because she has a right to know.
b. Tell her the truth because you have the legal obligation to do so.
c. Consult the ethics committee to help you make the decision.
d. Do not tell the patient's wife, but inform her that you will not tell her husband about the conversation you've just had.
e. Do not tell the patient's wife, but make an effort to encourage an open dialogue between her and her husband.

Complementary and Alternative Medicine

73. The practice where you are working cares for a wide variety of patients. Which of the following subgroups is most likely to explore and use complementary and alternative medicine (CAM)?

a. Children
b. College students
c. Men
d. Women
e. The elderly

74. Traditional therapies have offered limited benefit to a 55-year-old woman who suffers from migraine headaches, and she asks you about alternative therapies. She currently takes 325 mg of enteric-coated aspirin a day, and paroxetine, 20 mg daily. Which of the following has the lowest risk of toxicity or harm?

a. St. John's wort
b. Megavitamins
c. Macrobiotic diet
d. Ginkgo biloba
e. Acupuncture

75. You know that many of your patients have tried CAMs, but also know that patients may not reveal this to their physicians. What percentage of patients that use CAM practices reveal this information to their conventionally trained physicians?

a. Less than 5%
b. Approximately 10%
c. Approximately 30%
d. Approximately 50%
e. More than 50%

76. Of those patients who use CAM, how many use it as their exclusive treatment modality?

a. Less than 5%.
b. Approximately 10%.
c. Approximately 30%.
d. Approximately 50%.
e. Most patients who use CAM practices use them exclusively.

77. You are working with a smoker who has failed several attempts to quit smoking. He decides to try hypnosis in an effort to finally quit. Which major domain of alternative medicine does this best fit under?

a. Alternative health care systems
b. Mind-body interventions
c. Biologically based therapies
d. Energy therapies
e. Bioelectromagnetics

Palliative Care

78. After a prolonged fight with colon cancer, your 68-year-old patient decides to forego further attempts at curative treatment and focus on palliative care. He has tried nonsteroidal anti-inflammatory agents and acetaminophen for management of his pain, but this has been ineffective. Which of the following would be the best initial pain-management regimen?

a. A steroid burst to get the pain under control then scheduled nonsteroidal anti-inflammatory medications to maintain pain control
b. A long-acting narcotic pain patch at the lowest dose that controls the pain
c. A short-acting narcotic on a scheduled basis, with the possibility of additional short-acting narcotics as needed for breakthrough pain control
d. A long-acting narcotic, with a short-acting narcotic as needed for breakthrough pain
e. A patient-controlled analgesia device using opioids

79. Your patient has terminal cancer with a life expectancy of less than 3 months. You are managing her chronic cancer pain with morphine sulfate. She has been stable for weeks, but is requiring increasing amounts of opiates to maintain pain control. Which of the following statements is true regarding this situation?

a. The patient's disease is progressing and you should increase her medication dosage.
b. The patient's disease is progressing and you should change medications.
c. The patient is developing tolerance and you should increase her medication.
d. The patient is developing tolerance and you should maintain the dosage of medication to avoid dependence.
e. The patient is developing tolerance and you should slowly withdraw medication.

80. You are caring for a 68-year-old man who, 1 month ago, developed a rash. The rash consisted of grouped vesicles on erythematous bases in a dermatomal pattern. You effectively treated the rash, but the patient complained of a persistent burning and itching pain in the same area as the rash. The pain is significant and keeps him from sleeping. What is the best approach for long-term pain management in this patient?

a. Nonsteroidal anti-inflammatory agents
b. Opiate analgesics
c. Steroids
d. Anticonvulsants
e. Selective serotonin reuptake inhibitors

81. You are caring for a 65-year-old man with lung cancer. He was diagnosed 4 months ago, and is not expected to live for more than 2 months. He is experiencing dyspnea. His chest x-ray shows progression of his cancer, and his pulse oximetry shows a room air oxygen saturation of 94%. Which of the following is most likely to relieve his symptoms?

a. Opioids
b. Nebulized morphine
c. Steroids
d. Benzodiazepines
e. Albuterol

82. You are caring for a 68-year-old man who has had colon cancer for 3 years. Therapies have been unsuccessful, and he has chosen palliative care only. He complains of excessive fatigue, feeling tired after minimal activity, and lacking energy to perform the activities of daily living. He denies depression, and feels he is handling his diagnosis well with the support of his family and friends. His laboratory evaluation is normal, except for mild anemia. Which of the following therapies would be most likely to help his symptoms?

a. Transfusion
b. Nutritional supplementation
c. Selective serotonin reuptake inhibitors
d. Sedative hypnotics
e. Psychostimulant like methylphenidate

83. You are treating a 60-year-old patient with end-stage ovarian cancer. You are concerned that she may be developing depression. Which of the following would be the most reliable symptom of depression in this patient?

a. Loss of appetite
b. Fatigue
c. Insomnia
d. Sadness
e. Anhedonia

84. You are caring for a 39-year-old woman who is dying of breast cancer. Her family wonders how to recognize the symptoms of impending death. Which of the following is a reliable sign that death is near in this patient?

a. Delirium
b. Desire to communicate with loved ones
c. Difficulty swallowing
d. Desire for favorite food
e. Increased attention to dates and time

85. You are making a home visit to a 68-year-old man with terminal cancer. His family says that his breathing seems to be labored. Upon evaluation, you know that this is the "death rattle" that often signals approaching death. Which of the following drugs would be most useful in controlling this symptom?

a. Atropine
b. Ketorolac
c. Lorazepam
d. Haloperidol
e. Thorazine

Gay, Lesbian, Bisexual, and Transgender Issues

86. A 19-year-old sexually active homosexual male asks you about his risk for hepatitis. He is currently asymptomatic and unsure of his immune status. Which of the following should you recommend?

a. Vaccination against hepatitis A only
b. Vaccination against hepatitis B only
c. Vaccine against hepatitis C only
d. Vaccinations against both hepatitis A and B
e. Vaccinations against both hepatitis B and C

87. A 26-year-old homosexual man presents with blood on the toilet paper when wiping. Examination of the anal mucosa reveals this:

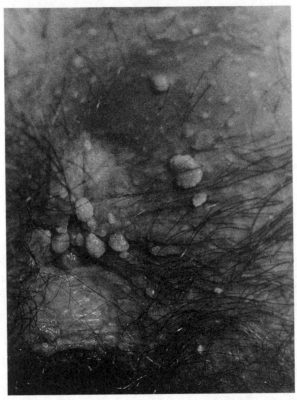

(Reproduced, with permission, from Wolff K, Johnson RA, Suurmond D. Fitzpatrick's Color Atlas and Synopsis of Clinical Dermatology, 5th ed. New York, NY: McGraw-Hill, 2005: 891.)

Which of the following statements is true regarding this condition?

a. This condition is rarely seen in men who are not immunocompromised.
b. The patient's physician should consider anal cytologic screening with a Papanicolaou (Pap) test.
c. The patient should be treated with intramuscular penicillin once a week for 3 weeks.
d. The patient should be treated with valciclovir.
e. The patient should be treated with one dose of azithromycin.

88. A 30-year-old gay male asks you about how his sexuality impacts his cancer risks. Which of the following statements most accurately reflect his risk for cancer?

a. Homosexual men have an increased rate of oral cancer.
b. Homosexual men have an increased rate of colon cancer.
c. Homosexual men have an increased rate of liver cancer.
d. Homosexual men have an increased rate of testicular cancer.
e. Homosexual men have an increased rate of anal cancer.

89. You are caring for a 42-year-old lesbian woman. She has recently left a 10-year monogamous relationship, and is concerned about her risk for vaginal and other infections, once she resumes sexual activity with a new partner. Which of the following is true regarding her concern?

a. The rate of sexually transmitted infections (STIs) among lesbians is less than the rate in heterosexual women.
b. The rate of genital warts is higher in lesbians than in heterosexual women.
c. The rate of bacterial vaginosis is higher in lesbians than in heterosexual women.
d. The rate of genital herpes is higher in lesbians than in heterosexual women.
e. Sexually active lesbians have a lower prevalence of HIV than women who have sex exclusively with men.

90. You are caring for a 40-year-old lesbian with no family history of breast cancer. She asks you about her risk of having breast cancer. Which of the following is true regarding breast cancer among lesbian women?

a. Breast cancer rates do not differ between lesbians and heterosexual women.
b. Breast cancer rates are higher among lesbians because of nonparity.
c. Breast cancer rates are higher among lesbians because of obesity.
d. Breast cancer rates are higher among lesbians because of alcohol and tobacco use.
e. Breast cancer rates are lower among lesbians because they generally use oral contraceptives less.

91. You are caring for a 25-year-old lesbian. She asks you about Pap testing in lesbian women. Which of the following is true about cervical cancer screening in this population?

a. Lesbians do not need Pap testing.
b. Lesbians do not need Pap testing, except if they are smokers.
c. Lesbians need Pap testing, but less frequently than heterosexual women.
d. Lesbians should be screened for cervical cancer at the same intervals that are recommended for heterosexual women.
e. Lesbians should be screened for cervical cancer more frequently than heterosexual women.

92. You are taking the complete history of a patient new to your office. The patient is dressed as a woman, but is biologically male. Further history reveals that the patient takes female hormones and is considering sexual reassignment surgery. What term most specifically describes this person?

a. Cross dresser
b. Bigender
c. Transvestite
d. Transsexual
e. Transgender

Doctor-Patient Issues

Answers

52. The answer is e. *(South-Paul, pp 641-646.)* Studies have shown that physicians often interrupt patients before they completely express their concerns. Physicians who do this and control the interview with directive questions often miss valuable and important information. These behaviors result in an incomplete clinical picture and collection of inaccurate information. Information is also lost when physicians use medical jargon. Patients frequently believe they understand the jargon, but are often incorrect. Involving the patient in his/her treatment plan is important, but that does not lead to the collection of accurate information. The use of closed-ended questions limits the patients' ability to fully describe their concerns. Communication is enhanced and accuracy is improved when physicians use open-ended questions, allow patients to fully answer questions before interrupting, and avoid technical or medical jargon.

53. The answer is b. *(South-Paul, pp 641-646.)* Dealing with the angry patient is challenging. A natural response to anger is defensiveness, but this can escalate the situation. The best approach is for the physician to first recognize the anger, acknowledge it, try to understand it, and respond to it. If a physician senses that a patient is angry, but the patient has not volunteered this information, it is important to explore the anger. If the patient seems very upset, it may make him/her angrier if the provider minimizes the situation by saying something like, "you seem a little upset." If a patient is extremely angry, choose words that seem to match the intensity of his/her feelings. In some instances anger is displaced, and may be truly directed at the disease process or illness. In that case, the appropriate response is empathy. However, in this setting, the anger is likely a response to the wait time that the patient has endured, and is less likely to be displaced. Placing the blame on your previous personal situation should be avoided—your patient likely will be empathetic to your situation, but it will not help meet his/her needs. It is important not to blame lateness on prior patients, even if that is the reason for the delay. It may make the current patient feel less important than the previous one. Apologizing for the delay may be appropriate, but the most patient-centered response would be to acknowledge what the patient appears to be feeling.

54. The answer is e. *(South-Paul, pp 641-646.)* Adherence is a complex issue for physicians and patients. In patients who do not adhere to their doctors' advice, the reasons usually relate to the patients' beliefs, goals and expectations. Asking the patient if he takes his medications is unlikely to yield accurate information, as the answer to this question is often an automatic "yes." However, patients will give accurate information about adherence about 80% of the time if the physician asks well-framed questions. By asking specific questions about names, dosages, and times, the physician will be more likely to elicit information about compliance. Another tactic may be to give permission for admitting noncompliance by saying something like, "Some of my patients find it difficult to remember to take their medications. Does this ever happen to you?"

Performing pill counts, measuring serum blood levels, and evaluating outcomes have not been shown in the medical literature to be effective measures of compliance.

55. The answer is a. *(South-Paul, pp 641-646.)* When motivating a patient to comply with a treatment regimen, it is important to explore their reasons for noncompliance. Once that is accomplished, the provider and patient should come to agreement on how to proceed. In this process, the physician can correct misconceptions, refer the patient to a trusted source of information, explore options, or suggest alternatives. Fear is not an effective motivator in most cases. Therefore, pointing out consequences of not following advice, or bringing up images of suffering patients is not effective. While empathy is appropriate to enhance the doctor-patient relationship, it is not always an effective motivational tool. Providing data often does not help, as patients do not see themselves as numbers and often do not understand how to apply the statistics to their situation. Patients are more likely to comply if you point out the positive results that can be expected by following your advice.

56. The answer is b. *(South-Paul, pp 641-646.)* When giving a patient bad news, attention should be given to the setting. Ensure the room is private and free of interruptions and that you have enough time for the visit. Some patients may want someone else present, but others may not. When suspicious that a test result may be positive, the physician may consider asking the patient in advance if they would like a support person present when reviewing the results. By beginning the session with an inquiry of the patient's knowledge, you are effectively giving the diagnosis without allowing the patient to prepare. Using a "warning" statement allows the patient to mentally prepare for the upcoming information. The discussion of treatment goals and options will likely overwhelm the patient, and should be deferred to a subsequent session. The physician should be hopeful, but realistic. Ensuring a cure for the disease may be detrimental.

57. The answer is c. *(South-Paul, pp 641-646.)* Patients commonly believe their physician does not give them enough information. However, studies show that patients often misunderstand or do not remember the information that physicians give them. Techniques physicians can employ to improve recall include simplification, repetition, giving specific information, and checking for understanding. Patients generally appreciate this, and generally do not feel this is patronizing. Nonverbal techniques including decreased interpersonal distance, more eye contact, and leaning toward the patient have been shown to improve recall. Patients are more likely to make behavior change if presented with several choices. However, too many options may be overwhelming. Statements like, "Your options are . . ." and "Which option do you think will be best for you?" are often helpful.

58. The answer is d. *(South-Paul, pp 647-654.)* Health, illness, and treatment are strongly influenced by cultural contexts. Although those trained in the United States have illness and treatment concepts based on biomedicine, many in other cultures define illness in other ways with different disease classifications and responses to them. Asking a patient of another culture what she thinks may be causing the problem and about treatment options demonstrates respect for the patient and her culture. Having Americanized relatives try to convince her would not respect her cultural beliefs. Pretending to understand her cultural and health beliefs may cause resentment. Continuing to focus on the biomedical model does not respect the cultural aspects of disease. Using an interpreter, while often necessary, does not address the underlying cultural issue.

59. The answer is a. *(South-Paul, pp 647-654.)* Recommendations for working with a medically trained interpreter include:

- Greet the patient in his/her own language if possible.
- Introduce yourself to everyone present.
- Arrange the seats in a triad, and address the patient.
- Speak clearly, in a normal voice volume.
- Use common terms and simple language structure.
- Express one idea at a time and pause for the interpreter.
- Expect the interpreter to use first person singular, verbatim translation.
- Consider multiple meanings to nonverbal gestures.
- Ask the same questions in different ways if you get inconsistent or unconnected responses.
- Ask the interpreter to explain, but do not place the interpreter in the middle of conflicts.

60. The answer is d. (*South-Paul, pp 647-654.*) It is important to remember that physicians tend to focus on the biological process of disease, while patients focus on the illness experience, regardless of culture. Physicians should be familiar with the medically related cultural norms of the patients residing in their community, but also need to recognize that the norms are not stereotypical statements about all people from that culture. Individuals within groups may have different practices. As such, the most appropriate approach would be to Listen to your patient's perspective, Explain your plan, Acknowledge similarities and differences, Recommend an action and Negotiate a plan (LEARN).

61. The answer is c. (*South-Paul, pp 655-663.*) In the 2000 census, Native Americans made up only 0.7% of the population, but the prevalence of diabetes, obesity, alcoholism, and suicide is substantially higher in this population than others.

62. The answer is b. (*South-Paul, pp 655-663.*) Homelessness results in poor health status and high service use among children. Homeless children experience a higher number of acute illness symptoms, including fever, ear infections, diarrhea, and asthma exacerbations. Unfortunately, the emergency department tends to be a primary source of care for this group, and visits are higher among this population.

63. The answer is a. (*South-Paul, pp 655-663.*) Interestingly, the uninsured have lower rates of chronic health conditions as compared with the insured population. The reason for his may reflect the fact that uninsured people often work in physically demanding jobs with fewer benefits. Those with chronic debilitating disease are unable to continue working and may go on public assistance. The uninsured have a higher mortality rate, poorer general health status, and poorer mental health status. Uninsured children have similar rates of chronic disease and limitations of activity when compared with insured children.

64. The answer is d. (*South-Paul, pp 655-663.*) At each age of the lifespan African Americans, Hispanics, and Native Americans have a higher mortality rate than whites. Only Asians, in aggregate, average lower mortality rates than whites.

65. The answer is c. (*South-Paul, pp 655-663.*) Mental health disparities have existed in minority cultures for decades. The practice of psychiatry is heavily influenced by culture, perceptions of illness, and appropriate treatment. Mental health disorders are diagnosed more commonly in non-whites than in their white counterparts. This may be partly due to poor validation of the Diagnostic and Statistical Manual of Mental Disorder (Fourth Edition) *DSM-(IV)* and the unfamiliarity of many psychiatrists with culturally defined syndromes and folk healing systems. Screening is difficult because there is a lack of language-specific validated instruments, and interpreters may miss nuances in translation. This leads to misdiagnosis. Many cultures express distress as somatic complaints. It is well-known that feeling accepted in society, increased acculturation and a good transition to the new culture decreases mental health issues, while increased resistance to new culture lowers mental health.

66. The answer is a. (*Brennan, pp 243-246.*) There are three fundamental principles of professionalism. The first is the principle of primacy of patient welfare. This is based on a dedication to serving the interest of the patient, and deals with doing no harm. This is the principle violated in the question. The principle of patient autonomy involves empowering patients to make informed decisions regarding their treatment. The principle of social justice involves working to eliminate discrimination in health care. Professional competence is a professional responsibility, not a fundamental principle, and deals with commitment to lifelong learning and maintaining medical knowledge. Patient honesty is also a responsibility, and deals with informed consent and acknowledging medical errors.

67. The answer is d. *(Brennan, pp 243-246.)* Improving quality of care is a professional responsibility that all physicians must embrace. The commitment involves maintaining clinical competence, but also working collaboratively with other professionals to reduce medical error. Honesty deals with informed consent and acknowledging errors with patients. Maintaining appropriate relationships deals with not exploiting patient relationships. Commitment to maintaining trust involves managing conflict of interests.

68. The answer is b. *(Brennan, pp 243-246.)* Fundamental principles of professionalism (patient welfare, patient autonomy, and social justice) are central to the job of being a physician. Despite the fact that the patient would not be harmed if the student practiced the procedure, the patient was not given the chance to make an informed decision about participating in this activity. Therefore, autonomy has been violated.

69. The answer is e. *(Brennan, pp 243-246.)* When other people can hear, it is important to ensure patient confidentiality. Appropriate safeguards should be applied to the disclosure of any patient information, including sensitive information regarding diagnosis and treatment. Despite the fact that the patient may do better on the new regimen, it is not appropriate to discuss it in the presence of others not associated with the patient's case.

70. The answer is e. *(Brennan, pp 243-246.)* The principle of patient autonomy requires physicians to be honest with their patients about treatment options, as well as the options if treatment is refused. Patient's decisions about their care are paramount, as long as those decisions are made competently. However, in difficult cases such as this one, it is recommended that legal counsel be obtained.

71. The answer is a. *(Brennan, pp 243-246.)* Convincing a patient to change his mind disregards patient autonomy. Consulting an ethics committee and evaluating the patient's competency are unnecessary at this point. Discharging the patient from your practice for disagreeing with you would be inappropriate.

72. The answer is e. *(Brennan, pp 243-246.)* Patient confidentiality demands that you maintain safeguards related to the disclosure of patient information. This is dictated by the patient, even if the wife is the other person in the communication triad.

73. The answer is d. *(South-Paul, pp 549-557.)* Rates of CAM use are significant in all populations, but studies have shown that women are consistently more likely to explore and use CAM. Women are frequently central to the health care decisions made in a family, and when surveyed, 49% of women have used CAM. Other surveys have shown that 50% of patients with cancer or HIV will use unconventional medical practices at some point during their illness. CAM is gaining public interest, and becoming increasingly popular in the United States. In fact, between 1990 to 1996, the amount spend on CAM rose from $14 billion to $27 billion.

74. The answer is e. *(South-Paul, pp 549-557.)* When discussing CAM, physicians should help patients make informed choices. Many practices, including acupuncture, biofeedback, homeopathy, and meditation are low risk if used by competent practitioners. Many herbal substances can interact with traditional medications and cause harm. St. John's wort can cause serotonin syndrome when used with a selective serotonin reuptake inhibitor like paroxetine. Megavitamins carry with them the risk of toxicity. Special diets, including the macrobiotic diet (high complex carbohydrate, low-fat, vegetarian diet) may have harmful effects, including undesirable changes in weight and bowel habits. Ginkgo biloba has antiplatelet effects, and may cause bleeding when taken with aspirin.

75. The answer is c. *(South-Paul, pp 549-557.)* There is a major communication gap between physicians and the public regarding CAM practices. More than 70% of patients who use CAM do not reveal this to their conventional physicians. Often, they fear reprisal from their physician. If physicians are open to hearing about therapies, and react to the knowledge in a nonjudgmental fashion, patients will feel more comfortable sharing the information, and patient care will be improved. Practitioners should recommend the "P's"—protect from risk, permit use, promote discussion, and partner with patients.

76. The answer is a. *(South-Paul, pp 549-557.)* The overwhelming majority of patients who use CAM use it as an adjunct to more traditional western therapies. Less than 5% use CAM exclusively. In general, patients who use CAM do not harbor an "antiscience" sentiment. Patients who use CAM do not include a disproportionate number of uneducated, poor or mentally ill representatives. Often, the attraction to CAM is philosophical, and is consistent with the patient's overall health beliefs.

77. The answer is b. *(South-Paul, pp 549-557.)* The National Center for Complementary and Alternative Medicine, National Institutes of Health, has grouped CAM modalities into several domains. Mind-body interventions include things like meditation, hypnosis, guided imagery, prayer, and mental healing. Alternative health care systems include Ayurvedic medicine, chiropractic medicine, and traditional Chinese medicine. Biologically based therapies include herbal therapies, special diets, and specific biologic therapies (like shark cartilage or bee pollen). Energy therapies include Qigong and Reiki therapy, and bioelectromagnetics include magnet therapy.

78. The answer is c. *(South-Paul, pp 558-565.)* The World Health Organization published guidelines for pain control in 1996. These guidelines have been well-studied and lead to effective pain control in most situations. In general, failing nonopioid pain control should lead to the use of opioid analgesics. Steroids have limited, if any, use in chronic cancer pain. Fentanyl patches, even at the lowest dose, may be excessive in opiate naïve patients, and should never be used alone. Most start with immediate-release morphine sulfate to determine a baseline need. This can be converted to sustained release quickly, and titrated based on pain control. Patient-controlled analgesia devices have an important role, but require intravenous or subcutaneous administration, and should not be used first-line, unless pain is extreme.

79. The answer is a. *(South-Paul, pp 558-565.)* Managing chronic cancer pain with opiates is often concerning for physicians. Many fear addiction and are concerned about causing harm. It is important to remember that there is no specific limit to opioid dose, and medications should be titrated to pain control or development of significant side effects. Fear of addiction should not hinder the use of opiates in this situation. Addiction is a rare occurrence in patients with terminal illness, especially in patients without a history of drug abuse. In patients on previously steady doses, dose escalation generally means the disease is progressing rather than tolerance. Tolerance, like addiction, is rarely seen in these patients.

80. The answer is d. *(South-Paul, pp 674-689.)* Neuropathic pain, like that described from shingles in this question, frequently requires opioids in the short term, but often requires the use of other medications for long-term relief. Commonly used medications includes tricyclic antidepressants, anticonvulsants (valproic acid, carbamazepine, gabapentin are the most common), and antihistamines. The data on using selective serotonin reuptake inhibitors are unconvincing.

81. The answer is a. *(South-Paul, pp 674-689.)* Dyspnea, like pain, is a subjective sensation. It can be present in the absence of hypoxia. Opioids can relieve breathlessness associated with advanced cancer by an unclear mechanism. Nebulized morphine isn't more effective than placebo. Steroids and albuterol are useful for dyspnea caused by bronchospasm, but that is unlikely in this case. Anxiolytics, like benzodiazepines and buspirone, may help if anxiety is a significant component, but that is usually expressed by patients as a feeling of "choking" or "suffocation."

82. The answer is e. *(South-Paul, pp 674-689.)* Excessive fatigue seen with end-stage cancer may result from direct tumor effects, paraneoplastic neuropathy, or tumor involvement of the CNS. It is often an effect of therapy. When no specific cause is apparent, as in this question, therapy is difficult. Transfusion is unlikely to be beneficial given his hemoglobin level. There is no evidence that the patient has a nutritional deficit, and supplementation may not be helpful. Although fatigue is frequently seen as a symptom of depression and may respond to selective serotonin reuptake inhibitor therapy, in this case it is unlikely. Sleeping pills would not help unless insomnia is the cause. A short course of steroids or a psychostimulant can increase energy and improve mood.

83. The answer is e. *(South-Paul, pp 674-689.)* It is commonly assumed that all patients with cancer are, and should be, depressed. Physicians often do not recognize depression because they feel they would be depressed in the same situation. While neurovegetative symptoms are a compelling indication of depression in the physically healthy patient, they may be less reliable for the diagnosis of depression in patients with advanced cancer. Loss of appetite may be due to therapy, fatigue may be due to insomnia from untreated pain. Sadness may be appropriate, given the diagnosis. Anhedonia is a useful, if not the most useful symptom to monitor. Also helpful are hopelessness, guilt, and a wish to die.

84. The answer is c. *(South-Paul, pp 674-689.)* As death approaches, there are several signs that portend its arrival. Delirium may be a result of medication, and by itself is not a good indicator. Other indicators are:

- Remaining bedbound
- Confusion
- Cool and mottled extremities
- The "death rattle"
- Decreased hearing/vision
- Difficulty swallowing
- Decreased conversation
- Decreased oral intake
- Disorientation to time
- Drowsiness progressing to somnolence for extended periods
- Dry mouth
- Hallucinations
- Increased distance from all but a few intimate others
- Decreased attention span
- Profound weakness

85. The answer is a. *(South-Paul, pp 674-689.)* Atropine can decrease secretions and help the "death rattle." Other medications that may be useful include scopolamine, glycopyrolate, mycosamine, or morphine. Ketorolac may help pain, lorazepam may help restlessness, haloperidol and thorazine may help agitation and hallucinations, both of which are also symptoms of impending death.

86. The answer is d. *(South-Paul, pp 664-673.)* The unique health needs of gay men may often be overlooked by physicians, especially if not alert to appropriate and sympathetic sexual history-taking. Since hepatitis A is transmitted orally/fecally, and many gay men participate in oral/anal sexual activity, vaccination against hepatitis A is appropriate. Since hepatitis B is transmitted through blood and body fluids, and sometimes by anal intercourse, hepatitis B vaccination is indicated. There is no vaccination against hepatitis C.

87. The answer is b. *(South-Paul, pp 664-673.)* The picture above represents infection with human papillomavirus (HPV). The prevalence of this infection is high, and in one study, 65.9% of HIV negative gay men were found to be positive for anal HPV. Penicillin treats syphilis, valciclovir treats herpes, and azithromycin treats *Chlamydia* and gonorrhea (2 g of azithromycin are needed to treat gonorrhea and *Chlamydia*). Men infected with HPV have been shown to have anal dysplasia, and cytologic screening should be considered for gay men positive for HPV.

88. The answer is e. *(South-Paul, pp 664-673.)* The increase in anal cancer in homosexual men is due to the increase in anal HPV infection seen in the gay male population. This is even seen in men without HIV. The other cancers listed do not seem to have an increased incidence in gay men.

89. The answer is c. *(South-Paul, pp 664-673.)* Generally, lesbians are felt to be at less risk for STIs than heterosexual women. However, most studies indicate comparable rates of STIs between lesbians and heterosexual women. Interestingly, the type of STI is different. Genital warts and genital herpes are more common in heterosexuals, with bacterial vaginosis being more common in lesbians. There is a mistaken belief that lesbians are not at risk for acquiring HIV. However, it has been shown that sexually active lesbians have a *higher* prevalence of HIV than women who have sex exclusively with men.

90. The answer is a. *(South-Paul, pp 664-673.)* Survey data from almost 12,000 women found no difference in breast cancer rates between lesbians and heterosexual women. Intuitively, one would think cancer rates would be higher because of nulliparity and higher rates of obesity. However, well-designed prospective studies have not been done to establish that as a fact.

91. The answer is d. *(South-Paul, pp 664-673.)* Cervical cancer may be less prevalent in women who have never had heterosexual vaginal intercourse, however, even in women reporting that they have never had sex with a man, up to 20% were found to have HPV DNA. Also, many physicians assume self-reported lesbians to have never had sex with a man, when some studies have reported that up to 79% of lesbians have reported having sex with a male in the past. Therefore, physicians should follow Pap smear screening guidelines in place for all women regardless of the woman's reported sexuality.

92. The answer is d. *(South-Paul, pp 664-673.)* Transgender is an umbrella term describing a group of people who cross culturally defined gender categories. Cross dressers wear the clothes of the other gender, but may not completely identify with that gender. Bigender individuals identify with both genders. Transvestites dress as another gender, but have not considered surgery. Transexuals wish to change their sex, and have considered or undertaken surgery.

Acute Complaints

Questions

93. You are evaluating a 41-year-old man in your office who reports abdominal pain. He says the pain began suddenly and is located in the right lower quadrant. He describes the pain as "gnawing" and it seems to get worse after eating. He has vomited twice since the pain began. Which historical feature would lead you toward an emergent evaluation?

a. The pain's location in the right lower quadrant
b. The fact that the pain began suddenly
c. The description of the pain
d. The fact that it is worse after eating
e. The fact that it is associated with emesis

94. A 42-year-old woman presents to your office complaining of abdominal pain. She describes upper abdominal pain that radiates to her scapula. For which of the following is this a classic description?

a. Acute appendicitis
b. Pancreatitis
c. Gallbladder disease
d. Esophageal spasm
e. Gastroesophageal reflux disease (GERD)

95. An 80-year-old man presents with mild, crampy, bilateral lower quadrant pain, decreased appetite, and low-grade fever for about 48 hours. Which of the following is the most likely diagnosis?

a. Small-bowel obstruction
b. Appendicitis
c. Constipation
d. Irritable-bowel syndrome (IBS)
e. Pancreatitis

96. While performing an abdominal examination on a 42-year-old woman in your office, she suddenly stops inspiratory effort during deep palpation of the right upper quadrant. Of which of the following problems is this most suggestive?

a. Hepatitis
b. Gallstones
c. Cholecystitis
d. Pancreatitis
e. Right-sided renal calculi

97. A 56-year-old is complaining of gnawing abdominal pain in the center of her upper abdomen associated with a sensation of hunger. She has a long history of alcohol abuse, and notes darker stool over the last 3 weeks. Which of the following is the most likely cause of her illness?

a. Alcoholism
b. Nonsteroidal anti-inflammatory drug (NSAID) abuse
c. *Helicobacter pylori* infection
d. Gallstones
e. Gastroparesis

98. A 26-year-old man presents complaining of heartburn. He also complains of regurgitation, belching, and occasional dry cough. His symptoms are worse when he is lying down. He denies melena, weight loss, or dysphagia. What is the appropriate next step, if you suspect GERD in this patient?

a. Treat with H_2-receptor antagonists, a proton pump inhibitor, or a prokinetic agent and evaluate the response
b. Obtain a barium swallow
c. Obtain a computed tomographic (CT) scan of the abdomen with oral and intravenous (IV) contrast
d. Obtain an ultrasound of the abdomen
e. Perform an esophagogastroduodenoscopy (EGD)

99. You are seeing a 75-year-old patient with complaints of heartburn, regurgitation, and belching. You suspect GERD. Which symptom, if present, would necessitate a referral for an upper endoscopy?

a. Pain radiating to the back
b. Dysphagia
c. Chronic use of NSAIDs for coexisting arthritis
d. Bloating
e. Nausea

100. A 44-year-old woman is admitted to the hospital for acute right upper quadrant pain consistent with biliary colic. Her symptoms have been present for 4 hours, and she also has fever and a positive Murphy sign. She has a history of asymptomatic gallstones, identified incidentally several years ago. Her laboratory evaluation is as follows:

White blood cell (WBC):	17.5 K/µL (H) with a left shift
Aspartate aminotransferase (AST):	88 U/L (H)
Alanine aminotransferase (ALT):	110 U/L (H)
Alkaline phosphatase:	330 U/L (H)
Bilirubin (total):	3.2 mg/dL (H)

What would the next test of choice be?

a. Ultrasound of the abdomen
b. CT scan of the abdomen
c. Magnetic resonance imaging (MRI) of the abdomen
d. Endoscopic retrograde cholangiopancreatography (ERCP)
e. Cholescintigraphy

101. You are seeing a patient who reports the abrupt onset of deep epigastric pain with radiation to the back associated with nausea, vomiting, sweating, and weakness. On examination, his abdomen is distended and tender in the epigastric area. Which of the following is the most common cause of this condition?

a. Gallstones
b. Alcohol abuse
c. Iatrogenic cause
d. Idiopathic cause
e. Hyperlipidemia

102. You are concerned about pancreatitis in a 44-year-old woman with acute symptoms. Which of the following laboratory tests is most specific for pancreatitis?

a. WBC count
b. Amylase
c. Lipase
d. AST
e. ALT

103. You are seeing a 53-year-old man who was hospitalized for pancreatitis. His admission laboratory studies include a WBC count of 18,000/mm³, glucose of 153 mg/dL, lactate dehydrogenase (LDH) of 254 IU/L, and AST of 165 U/L. According to Ranson criteria, which of these factors suggest a poor prognosis in this patient?

a. Age
b. WBC count
c. Glucose
d. LDH
e. AST

104. You are evaluating a patient new to your practice who is complaining of abdominal pain. The pain has been present on and off for more than 2 years, and has been present more often than not for the preceding 6 months. She reports that her pain is related to defecation and is associated with diarrhea. Which of the following is true regarding diagnostic testing for her condition?

a. A normal complete blood count (CBC) is necessary for diagnosis
b. A normal erythrocyte sedimentation rate (ESR) is necessary for diagnosis
c. A colonoscopy is necessary for diagnosis
d. Normal stool cultures are necessary for diagnosis
e. No tests are necessary to diagnose this condition

105. A 65-year-old man presents to you complaining of abdominal pain. His pain is associated with anorexia, bloating, nausea, and vomiting. He is afebrile and denies fever. On examination, his abdomen appears distended, and he has absent bowel sounds. Abdominal percussion produces tympani. What would his abdominal x-ray most likely show?

a. Fecalith in the right lower quadrant
b. Free intraperitoneal air
c. Stool throughout the colon
d. Proximally dilated loops of bowel
e. Stones in the right upper quadrant

106. You are seeing a 46-year-old man who reports 3 months of discomfort centered around his upper abdomen. It is associated with heartburn, frequent belching, bloating, and occasional nausea. What is the most likely result that will be found after workup for these symptoms?

a. Peptic ulcer disease
b. GERD
c. Gastric cancer
d. Gastroparesis
e. No cause is likely to be identified

107. You are caring for a 26-year-old generally healthy woman. She is sexually active and currently in a monogamous relationship. You recently completed her annual examination. Her Pap smear reports "atypical squamous cells of undetermined significance." Human papillomavirus (HPV) testing was negative. Which of the following is the most appropriate next step?

a. Repeat the Pap smear immediately.
b. Treat the patient with metronidazole and repeat the Pap smear when the course of antibiotics is finished.
c. Repeat the Pap smear in 4 to 6 months.
d. Repeat the Pap smear in 1 year.
e. Perform colposcopy.

108. You are caring for a 24-year-old generally healthy woman. She is sexually active and currently in a monogamous relationship, using oral contraceptives. You recently completed her annual examination. Her Pap smear reports "atypical squamous cells of undetermined significance." HPV testing was positive. Which of the following is the most appropriate next step?

a. Repeat the Pap smear immediately.
b. Repeat the Pap smear in 4 to 6 months.
c. Repeat the Pap smear in 1 year.
d. Perform colposcopy.
e. Treat the patient with imiquimod (Aldara) and repeat the Pap smear after the treatment is complete.

109. You are caring for a 40-year-old obese woman with mild hypertension. She is sexually active with her husband of 16 years, and had a tubal ligation after her son was born 5 years ago. One year ago, her Pap smear reported "atypical squamous cells of undetermined significance." HPV testing at your institution was unavailable. You repeated the Pap smear at 4 months and 8 months after the initial sample was taken. Both of those samples were normal. Which of the following is the most appropriate next step?

a. Repeat the Pap smear immediately.
b. Repeat the Pap smear in 4 to 6 months.
c. Repeat the Pap smear in 1 year.
d. Perform colposcopy.
e. Treat the patient with fluconazole (Diflucan) and repeat the Pap smear after the treatment is complete.

110. You are caring for a 28-year-old generally healthy woman. She is currently not sexually active, but has had multiple partners in the past. You recently completed her annual examination. Her Pap smear reports "atypical squamous cells of undetermined significance, favor low-grade squamous intraepithelial lesion." Which of the following is the most appropriate next step?

a. Repeat the Pap smear immediately
b. Repeat the Pap smear in 4 to 6 months
c. Repeat the Pap smear in 1 year
d. Perform colposcopy
e. Perform endometrial biopsy

111. You are caring for a 34-year-old generally healthy woman. She is sexually active and currently in a monogamous relationship with her husband, using oral contraceptives. You recently completed her annual examination. Her Pap smear reports "atypical glandular cells," but does not specify if those cells are endocervical or endometrial in origin. She has not had any abnormal vaginal bleeding. Which of the following is the most appropriate next step?

a. Repeat the Pap smear immediately
b. Repeat the Pap smear in 4 to 6 months
c. Repeat the Pap smear in 1 year
d. Perform colposcopy
e. Perform endometrial biopsy

112. You are caring for a 46-year-old generally healthy woman. She is sexually active with her husband only. You recently completed her annual examination. Her Pap smear reports "atypical glandular cells" and are reported to be of endometrial origin. She does not report any abnormal vaginal bleeding. Which of the following is the most appropriate next step?

a. Repeat the Pap smear immediately
b. Repeat the Pap smear in 4 to 6 months
c. Repeat the Pap smear in 1 year
d. Perform colposcopy
e. Perform endometrial biopsy

113. An 18-year-old woman is seeing you for an evaluation of her fatigue. She also complains of exercise intolerance and reports an unusual desire to chew ice in the last couple of months. You suspect anemia, and a point-of-care hemoglobin test confirms this diagnosis. What is the most likely cause of her anemia?

a. Iron deficiency
b. Lead toxicity
c. Autoimmune disease
d. Vitamin B_{12} deficiency
e. Folic acid deficiency

114. A laboratory analysis of one of your patients reveals a microcytic anemia. The red cell distribution width (RDW) is normal. Which of the following is the most likely diagnosis?

a. Iron deficiency
b. Sideroblastic anemia
c. Thalassemia
d. Aplastic anemia
e. Chronic renal insufficiency

115. A 60-year-old man is being evaluated for fatigue, weakness, and exercise intolerance. Laboratory assessment reveals:

Hemoglobin:	9.1 mg/dL (L)
Serum iron:	46 µg/dL (L)
Ferritin:	9 ng/mL (L)
Total iron binding capacity (TIBC):	626 µg/dL (H)
Mean corpuscular volume (MCV):	76 fL (L)

What is the most common cause of this condition?

a. Blood loss
b. Poor nutrition
c. Inadequate absorption of iron
d. Chronic disease
e. Folic acid deficiency

116. You are caring for a 64-year-old woman with longstanding lupus. Her hemoglobin is 10.4 g/dL, and her mean corpuscular volume is 76 fL (L). Further laboratory analysis reveals a serum iron of 40 µg/dL (L), a total iron binding capacity of 188 µg/dL (L), and a ferritin of 333 ng/mL (H). Which of the following approaches is most appropriate to improve her anemia?

a. Oral iron therapy
b. Parenteral iron therapy
c. Erythropoietin therapy
d. Transfusion
e. Better control of her lupus

117. You are performing a presurgical clearance evaluation on a 44-year-old otherwise healthy African American male who is undergoing a laparoscopic cholecystectomy. His CBC is shown below:

Hemoglobin:	10.6 g/dL (L)
Mean corpuscular volume:	(MCV) 54 fL (L)
Red blood cell (RBC) count:	6.3 M/µL (H)
Red cell distribution width (RDW):	14.1 (NL)

What is the most appropriate step prior to surgery?

a. Oral iron replacement for 4 weeks, then recheck before surgery
b. Parenteral iron replacement for 4 weeks, then recheck before surgery
c. Transfusion
d. Hemoglobin electrophoresis
e. Erythropoietin

118. You are evaluating a 26-year-old woman with fatigue. She also complains of lightheadedness, some minor weight loss, and paresthesias in her hands and feet. On examination, her vital signs are normal, but you note pallor and glossitis. Laboratory evaluation reveals a hemoglobin of 9.8 g/dL (L) and a MCV of 102 fL (H). Which of the following would be most likely to treat her condition?

a. Diet rich in green leafy vegetables
b. Diet rich in iron
c. Vitamin B_{12} supplementation
d. Folic acid supplementation
e. Iron supplementation

119. A 68-year-old man complains of fatigue. He has a history of hypertension, well-controlled with hydrochlorothiazide. He's recently lost 30 lb on a high protein, low carbohydrate diet. He drinks two to three beers daily, and smokes 10 cigarettes daily. Laboratory evaluation reveals a macrocytic anemia and vitamin B_{12} deficiency. Which of the following is the most likely cause?

a. Side effects of hydrochlorothiazide
b. High-protein diet
c. Low-carbohydrate diet
d. Alcohol intake
e. Inadequate vitamin B_{12} absorption

120. A 3-year-old African American boy is brought in by his parents with inconsolable crying. He reports extreme pain in his hands and upper extremities. Laboratory evaluation reveals a hemoglobin of 8.2 mg/dL. His peripheral blood smear is as follows:

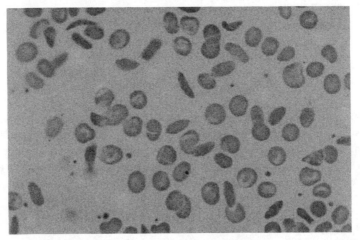

(Reproduced, with permission, from McPhee S, Papadakis M, and Tierney L. Current Medical Diagnosis and Treatment 2007, 46th ed. New York: McGraw-Hill, 2007.)

Which of the following measures would be most likely to reduce these events in the future?

a. Chronic use of analgesics
b. Adequate hydration
c. Immunization against streptococcal pneumonia
d. Monthly transfusions
e. Daily penicillin prophylaxis until the age of 5 years

121. You are seeing a 25-year-old male with a rash. It began as pink spots on his extremities, but the lesions have begun to coalesce and become purple in color. He recently returned from a hiking trip in the western mountains. Which of the following is the most likely cause?

a. Lyme disease
b. Rocky Mountain spotted fever
c. Tularemia
d. Brown recluse spider bite
e. Black widow spider bite

122. You are caring for a person who recently visited New England, and returns with a skin lesion suggestive of a bite. Which of the following arachnid-bourne illnesses is most likely to occur in the northeastern United States?

a. Lyme disease
b. Rocky Mountain spotted fever
c. Tularemia
d. Brown recluse spider bite
e. Chigger bites

123. You are seeing a patient who is complaining of an itching scalp. There are erythematous papules on her scalp, and you note small black bulbs at the bases of several hair follicles. Which of the following is the most likely cause?

a. Flea infestation
b. Bedbugs
c. Head lice
d. Scabies
e. Chigger bites

124. A 16-year-old camp counselor sees you to evaluate a severely pruritic rash. You note pruritic erythematous papules in between his fingers, on his wrists, and around his waist. For which of the following is this distribution characteristic?

a. Flea bites
b. Bedbugs
c. Body lice
d. Scabies
e. Chigger bites

125. While you are working in the emergency room, a 17-year-old patient presents with a cat bite. He was helping a neighbor get his cat out of a tree 3 hours ago, and was bitten on the forearm. On examination, you note erythema, a puncture wound with a jagged laceration but no tendon involvement. You irrigate the wound thoroughly. What additional therapy is indicated?

a. Hospitalization
b. Human rabies immune globulin
c. Amoxicillin/clavulanic acid
d. Clindamycin
e. Primary closure

126. A 20-year-old man presents to you 30 minutes after being stung by a bee on his right thigh. He was stung by a bee twice last year. The first sting caused a 3-cm by 3-cm area of erythema, induration, and pain around the sting site. The second sting caused a similar 5-cm by 7-cm area. When you examine him, he has an expanding 2-cm by 2-cm area of erythema, induration, and pain around the sting site on his thigh. He reports pruritis, fatigue, and some nausea, but denies dyspnea. Which of the following is true?

a. This is a typical local reaction, and should spontaneously resolve within hours.
b. This is a large local reaction, and the patient has minimal risk for the development of anaphylaxis upon subsequent exposure.
c. This is a large local reaction, and the patient is at significant risk for the development of anaphylaxis upon subsequent exposure.
d. This is considered a toxic systemic reaction, and increases his risk for anaphylaxis if he is exposed in the future.
e. This is considered a mild anaphylactic reaction.

127. A 15-year-old male comes to your office complaining of bilateral breast enlargement. He is otherwise healthy and on no medications. On examination, there is mildly tender palpable breast tissue bilaterally. The rest of his physical examination, including his testicular examination is normal. Which of the following is true?

a. No further workup is necessary.
b. Serum liver studies are needed to elucidate the cause.
c. Thyroid function assessment is needed to elucidate the cause.
d. Serum estradiol, testosterone, and leutinizing hormone levels are needed to elucidate the cause.
e. His serum chorionic gonadotropin level is likely to be elevated.

128. A 22-year-old woman is seeing her physician with complaints of breast pain. It is associated with her menstrual cycle and is described as a bilateral "heaviness" that radiates to the axillae and arms. Examination reveals groups of small breast nodules in the upper outer quadrants of each breast. They are freely mobile and slightly tender. Which of the following statements is most accurate?

a. The patient has bilateral fibroadenomas, and reassurance is all that is necessary.
b. The patient has bilateral fibroadenomas, and a mammogram is necessary for further evaluation.
c. The patient has bilateral fibrocystic changes, and reassurance is all that is necessary.
d. The patient has bilateral fibrocystic changes, and a mammogram is necessary for further evaluation.
e. The patient has bilateral mastitis, and antibiotic therapy is needed.

129. A 35-year-old woman presents to you concerned about a breast mass. Examination reveals no skin changes, diffusely nodular breasts bilaterally with a more dominant, firm, and nontender fixed nodule on the left side. The nodule is approximately 7 mm in size, in the upper outer quadrant of the left breast. Her mammogram is negative. Which of the following statements is true?

a. The patient should be reassured and resume routine care.
b. The mass should be closely followed with repeat mammogram in 3 to 6 months.
c. The patient should undergo testing for breast cancer genetic mutations, and base further workup on the results.
d. The patient should be referred for an ultrasound and possible biopsy.
e. If clear amber fluid is aspirated from the mass, it is likely benign, and no further workup is necessary.

130. A 28-year-old woman comes to see you for a tender and erythematous area on her breast. She is nursing her 6-week-old son. You diagnose mastitis. Which of the following is true regarding this condition?

a. Restricting caffeine and methylxanthine may be efficacious.
b. Evening primrose oil has been shown to help with symptoms.
c. Applying ice several times a day will help relieve symptoms.
d. The patient should discontinue nursing.
e. Antibiotic therapy is indicated.

131. You are seeing a 36-year-old woman with a complaint of nipple discharge. Which of the following characteristics of the discharge is most suspicious for breast cancer?

a. Spontaneous discharge
b. Green discharge
c. Bilateral discharge
d. Discharge associated with menses
e. Bloody discharge

132. On screening physical examination of a 36-year-old woman, you find a single left breast mass. It is 1 cm in size, firm, smooth, and apparently fixed to the underlying tissue. You perform a mammogram which is characterized as BI-RADS 3. What does this most likely indicate?

a. The physician should continue routine screening at the usual intervals.
b. The physician should perform additional tests (spot compression mammogram, ultrasound) to evaluate the mass as soon as possible.
c. The physician should perform diagnostic mammogram of the left breast in 6 months.
d. Tissue diagnosis is needed.
e. The mass is almost certainly cancerous.

133. You are caring for a 32-year-old woman whose 38-year-old sister was recently diagnosed with breast cancer. She asks if she can be screened for breast cancer using MRI. Which of the following is true regarding MRI screening for breast cancer?

a. MRI is not sensitive enough to be used as a screening modality for breast cancer.
b. MRI should be used to screen for breast cancer in anyone with a first-degree relative who has had breast cancer.
c. MRI is seen as a valuable screening tool for those with breast cancer genetic mutations.
d. MRI should only be used to clarify a suspicious finding on mammogram.
e. MRI should only be used to clarify suspicious findings on ultrasound.

134. You are evaluating a 21-year-old woman with an erythematous, tender, and edematous hand. She reports that while playing with her cat 3 days ago, he bit her and punctured the skin. The area around the bite is inflamed, and there is a purulent discharge from the puncture site. Which of the following is the most likely infecting organism?

a. *Clostridium perfringens*
b. *Staphylococcus aureus*
c. *Streptococcus pyogenes*
d. *Pasteurella multocida*
e. *Haemophilus influenzae*

135. You are evaluating a 22-year-old male patient who has recently developed a red rash. He just returned from a 4-day skiing trip, where he and his friends used the hot tub at the ski lodge daily. On examination, you note red dome-shaped pustules involving the hair follicles. What is the most likely cause of his rash?

a. Streptococcal infection of the hair follicles
b. Staphylococcal infection of the hair follicles
c. Pseudomonal infection of the hair follicles
d. Tinea infection of the hair follicles
e. Candidal infection of the hair follicles

136. You are seeing a 14-year-old high school wrestler for a skin condition. About a week ago, he noted a patch of erythematous skin on his right thigh. The patch has enlarged since he first noted it, and the central part of the lesion seems to be crusting and flaking. He reports that it is mildly pruritic. You scrape the lesion and evaluate the shavings under the microscope using potassium hydroxide. You visualize the following:

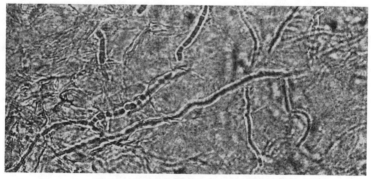

(Reproduced, with permission, from Wolff K, Johnson RA, Suurmond D. Fitzpatrick's Color Atlas and Synopsis of Clinical Dermatology, 5th ed. New York: McGraw-Hill, 2005: 689.)

Which of the following is the most likely diagnosis?

a. Tinea corporis
b. Tinea cruris
c. Pityriasis rosea
d. Nummular eczema
e. Impetigo

137. You are evaluating a 40-year-old male patient in the office who is complaining of chest pain. His father had a myocardial infarction at age 42, and the patient is quite concerned. Which characteristic, if included in the history, decreases the likelihood that his chest pain is cardiac in origin?

a. The pain is worse with inspiration
b. The pain radiates to his right arm
c. The pain radiates to his left arm
d. The pain is associated with nausea
e. The pain is associated with sweatiness

138. You are evaluating a 26-year-old female smoker who developed chest pain several hours ago. Her past history is unremarkable, and she takes no medications regularly. She reports the abrupt onset of nonexertional chest pain, associated with shortness of breath and cough. It seems to be worse when she is lying down. It was not brought on by trauma. Which of the following is the most likely origin of her pain?

a. Costochondritis
b. Asthma
c. Pulmonary embolus (PE)
d. Myocardial ischemia
e. Bronchitis

139. You are evaluating a 61-year-old man in the office who is complaining of chest pain. Given his history and risk factors, you are concerned about myocardial ischemia. Which of the following features, if present, would most reliably establish cardiac ischemia as a cause?

a. Relief of pain with nitroglycerine administration
b. Relief of pain with a "gastrointestinal (GI) cocktail" (viscous lidocaine and an antacid)
c. Relief of pain with cessation of activity
d. Relief of pain with eating
e. Relief of pain with sitting up and leaning forward

140. You are evaluating a 20-year-old man presenting to your office with the abrupt onset of chest pain. He has an unremarkable past medical history, but his father had his first myocardial infarction in his late 30s. On examination, he is thin and anxious-appearing. Other than tachycardia, his cardiac examination is normal. His lung examination reveals decreased breath sounds on the right, with hyperresonance to percussion. What is the best treatment for his condition?

a. Insertion of a chest tube
b. Antibiotic therapy
c. Bronchodilator therapy
d. Long-term anticoagulation
e. Immediately give 325 mg of aspirin, and transfer to an emergency room

141. A patient presents to your office in distress without an appointment. He is 23 years old and is complaining of severe chest pain. He reports a family history of coronary disease, complains of frequent "heartburn," and says he is recovering from a recent viral upper respiratory infection. He smokes one pack of cigarettes a day, and admits to illegal drug use in the past. On examination, his blood pressure is 138/90 mm Hg, his pulse is 126 beats per minute and regular, and he is diaphoretic. His examination is otherwise unremarkable. His electrocardiogram (ECG) shows myocardial ischemia. Which of his historical features are most suggestive that myocardial ischemia would be the cause of his symptoms?

a. Family history of coronary disease
b. History of "heartburn"
c. Recent viral upper respiratory infection
d. Smoking history
e. Drug use

142. A 45-year-old man with no significant past medical history presents to your office complaining of midsternal chest pain for 5 days. The pain is described as "sharp." On examination, the patient has normal breath sounds, but the pain increases with palpation. Which of the following is the most appropriate next step?

a. Obtain a chest x-ray
b. Obtain a CBC and blood cultures
c. Obtain an ECG
d. Treat with NSAIDs
e. Treat with a proton pump inhibitor

143. A 43-year-old woman with a history of well-controlled hypertension and diabetes presents to your office complaining of intermittent chest pain for the last 3 months. The last episode was 1 week ago, after climbing four flights of stairs at work. The pain was relieved with rest. An ECG in your office is shown below:

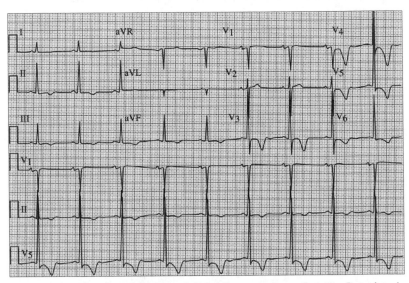

(Reproduced, with permission, from Ferry D. Basic Electrocardiography in Ten Days, *1st ed. New York: McGraw-Hill, 2001: 35.)*

She is currently asymptomatic. Which of the following is the most appropriate next step?

a. Reassure the patient and have her return if symptoms continue.
b. Reassure the patient, but increase her medication to ensure tight control of her blood pressure and glucose levels.
c. Admit the patient to the hospital for serial enzymes.
d. Obtain the patient's treadmill stress ECG.
e. Obtain the patient's treadmill stress echocardiogram.

144. You are evaluating a 75-year-old woman with diabetes and hyperlipidemia who is complaining of chest pain. She reports having occasional chest pain with exertion for years, but yesterday she reported syncope with the pain. On examination, she is afebrile with mildly elevated blood pressure. Cardiac auscultation demonstrates a harsh, rasping crescendo-decrescendo systolic murmur heard best at the second intercostal space at the right upper sternal border. Her carotid pulse is small and rises slowly. Which of the following is the most likely diagnosis?

a. PE
b. Aortic dissection
c. Left ventricular hypertrophy
d. Aortic stenosis
e. Mitral valve prolapse

145. You are evaluating a generally healthy 45-year-old man who is complaining of chest pain. His symptoms are typical for angina, and are relieved with rest. He is a nonsmoker, has no family history of heart disease, but has high cholesterol. His physical examination and ECG are normal. What is the most appropriate next step?

a. Exercise ECG testing
b. Exercise echocardiography
c. Pharmacologic myocardial perfusion imaging
d. Cardiac catheterization
e. Electron beam CT

146. One of your patients is undergoing stress testing for episodic chest pain. He is hypertensive and takes hydrochlorothiazide and metoprolol. Which of the following is the most appropriate advice to give this patient prior to undergoing the stress test?

a. Continue all medications as directed
b. Do not take either antihypertensive medication on the day of the test
c. Continue the metoprolol, but do not take hydrochlorozide at least 2 days before the test
d. Continue hydrocholothiazide, but withdraw the metoprolol at least 2 days before the test
e. Continue hydrochlorothiazide, but withdraw the metoprolol at least 6 days before the test

147. You are seeing a 44-year-old nonsmoker for an acute cough. The cough has been present for 4 days. He had a low-grade fever for the first 2 days, but that has resolved. He reports that the cough is worse at night, has become productive of yellow sputum, but there is no hemoptysis or shortness of breath. Which of the following is the most likely cause of the cough?

a. Pneumonia
b. Sinusitis with postnasal drip
c. Pertussis
d. Viral upper respiratory infection
e. Tuberculosis

148. A 33-year-old healthy nonsmoking man presents to you for evaluation of his chronic cough. He says the cough has been present for about 8 weeks. Initially, he went to an urgent care where he received antitussives and a bronchodilator. Those did not help, and he returned 1 week later and was given a course of azithromycin. His cough has continued to persist. His symptoms are worse when he lies down for sleep, and are associated with a sore throat. He has also noticed that when he drinks caffeine or alcohol, the cough seems to worsen. Which of the following is the most likely diagnosis?

a. GERD
b. Asthma
c. Side effect from a medication
d. Chronic bronchitis
e. Pertussis

149. You are treating a 52-year-old woman with a 40-pack/year history of smoking. She reports a productive cough that has been present for the last 3 to 4 months, beginning in the fall. She remembers having the same symptoms last year in the fall, and attributed it to a "cold that she just couldn't kick." She does not have fevers, reports mild dyspnea when walking up stairs, and denies hempotysis. Which of the following is the most likely diagnosis?

a. Irritation of airways from cigarette smoke
b. Chronic bronchitis
c. Postnasal drainage due to seasonal allergies
d. Lung cancer
e. Asthma

150. Four weeks ago, you treated a 22-year-old woman for acute bronchitis. Although she feels much better, the cough has persisted. She has used bronchodilators, antihistamines, and antitussives. Which of the following is the best course of treatment at this time?

a. A 10-day course of amoxicillin
b. A 5-day course of azithromycin
c. A steroid nasal spray
d. An NSAID
e. An oral steroid taper

151. You are seeing an 18-year-old man who has had a cough for 2 weeks. It started like a typical "cold," but has persisted. Over the last 3 days, the cough has come in "spasms" and he barely has time to catch his breath during the coughing episodes. Nasopharyngeal swab confirms the diagnosis of pertussis. Which of the following treatments is recommended?

a. A 10-day course of amoxicillin
b. A 10-day course of amoxicillin/clavulanate
c. A 7-day course of erythromycin
d. A 5-day course of azithromycin
e. A supportive therapy without antibiotics, but in isolation

152. You are seeing a 6-month-old boy whose mother reports that he has had diarrhea for almost 2 weeks. He has had four to six bowel movements a day, with a loose to liquid consistency. His mother stays at home with him and the child is not in daycare. His symptoms began after his young cousins visited for Christmas. Which of the following the most likely cause of his diarrhea?

a. Rotavirus
b. Norwalk virus
c. Giardiasis
d. *Salmonella*
e. Enterotoxigenic *Escherichia coli*

153. A 19-year-old man returned from a vacation in Mexico 1 day ago. He spent the last 3 days of his trip with loose, more frequent bowel movements that are continuing without resolution. He has not had bloody stool or fever. His examination is normal, except for mildly diffuse lower abdominal pain. Which of the following is the most likely cause of his diarrhea?

a. Rotavirus
b. Norwalk virus
c. Giardiasis
d. *Salmonella*
e. Enterotoxigenic *E coli*

154. You have diagnosed travelers' diarrhea in a 30-year-old otherwise healthy man who has recently returned from an African safari. Which of the following is the best empiric treatment option?

a. Erythromycin
b. Ciprofloxacin
c. Metronidazole
d. Doxycycline
e. Vancomycin

155. A 22-year-old healthy male sees you for "diarrhea." He reports frequent loose stools without bleeding. You determine that he likely has a virally mediated process and recommend supportive care. Which of the following dietary measures should you recommend?

a. The patient should fast until the diarrhea resolves.
b. The patient should not eat solids, but should drink an oral rehydrating solution.
c. The patient should drink milk.
d. The patient should drink fruit juice.
e. The patient can eat rice and potatoes.

156. A 33-year-old woman is seeing you with a chief complaint of "dizziness." Upon further characterization, she describes "unsteadiness" and a feeling that "her balance is off." Based on this description, which of the following terms should be used to characterize her complaint?

a. Vertigo
b. Orthostasis
c. Presyncope
d. Dysequilibrium
e. Lightheadedness

157. A 42-year-old woman is seeing you to follow up with a new complaint of "dizziness." She reports that symptoms first began several months ago. At that time, she reported a subjective hearing loss and a ringing in her left ear only. Symptoms were mild, and her physical examination was normal, so you elected to follow her. Since that time, her symptoms have progressed to include dizziness and some facial numbness. Which of the following is her most likely diagnosis?

a. Vestibular neuronitis
b. Benign positional vertigo
c. Acoustic neuroma
d. Meniere disease
e. Cerebellar tumor

158. In the evaluation of a 55-year-old man complaining of dizziness, you perform the Dix-Hallpike (Nylen-Barany) maneuver several times. You had the patient sit on the edge of the examining table and lie down suddenly with the head hanging 45° backward and turned to either side. With this maneuver, the vertigo was reproduced immediately, and symptoms did not lessen regardless of repetition. The direction of the nystagmus changed with changing the direction that the head is turned, and the symptoms were of mild intensity. Which of the following is the most likely cause of the vertigo?

a. Stroke
b. Vestibular neuronitis
c. Benign positional vertigo
d. Meinere disease
e. Acoustic neuroma

159. You are caring for a 26-year-old man with vertigo. You have diagnosed him with a peripheral vestibular disorder, and are considering treatment options. Which of the following would be the first-line therapy?

a. NSAIDs
b. Antihistamines
c. Antiemetics
d. Antibiotics
e. Benzodiazepines

160. You are evaluating a 56-year-old farmer who is complaining of dyspnea. His history includes being hospitalized for bronchiolitis as a young child leading to childhood asthma, and a history of pneumonia 2 years ago, for which he was also hospitalized. He has a 20-pack/year history of smoking. Which of the following increase his risk for having restrictive lung disease as the cause of his dyspnea?

a. A history of childhood bronchiolitis
b. A history of asthma
c. A smoking history
d. A recent history of pneumonia
e. His occupation as a farmer

161. You are seeing a 24-year-old male patient who reports feeling short of breath. He had an upper respiratory infection 3 weeks ago, but that resolved. Lately he has had progressive weakness, and yesterday began feeling short of breath. He is worse today. On examination, he has symmetric proximal leg muscle weakness with depressed deep tendon reflexes. His lung examination reveals decreased inspiratory volume without crackles or wheezes. Which of the following is his most likely diagnosis?

a. Parkinson disease
b. Amyotrophic lateral sclerosis
c. Lyme disease
d. Guillain-Barre syndrome
e. Psychogenic weakness and dyspnea

162. You are evaluating a 36-year-old woman with dyspnea. She reports a cough and some pleuritic chest pain. On examination, her temperature is 101°F, and you note egophony in the left lower lobe. Which of the following is the best treatment approach?

a. Reassurance
b. Bronchodilators
c. Antibiotics
d. Diuretics
e. Anticoagulants

163. You are evaluating a 71-year-old male patient with the complaint of shortness of breath. It mainly occurs with exertion. He also complains of fatigue, and needing to sleep propped up on two pillows. On physical examination, you note a large apical impulse and jugular venous distension (JVD). He has fine crackles in the bases of both lungs with decreased breath sounds. Which of the following would be the most appropriate treatment?

a. Bronchodilators
b. Antibiotics
c. Steroids
d. Anticoagulants
e. Diuretics

164. You are seeing a 3-year-old child whose mother says she is having trouble breathing. This is her third episode of difficulty breathing in the last year. On examination, you note nasal flaring and sternal retractions with accessory muscle use. You auscultate expiratory wheezes bilaterally. Which of the following is the most likely diagnosis?

a. Bronchiolitis
b. Asthma
c. Pneumonia
d. Ventricular septal defect
e. Valvular disease

165. You are evaluating a 69-year-old woman with a history of asthma and ischemic cardiomyopathy who is complaining of dyspnea. You are not sure if her symptoms are related to asthma or congestive heart failure (CHF), and you order a b-type natriuretic peptide to help in her evaluation. The level is found to be 76 pg/mL (normal is 0-100 pg/mL). Which of the following is most correct regarding the interpretation of this laboratory value?

a. The probability that her symptoms are related to CHF is near zero.
b. The probability that her symptoms are related to CHF is low.
c. The probability that her symptoms are related to CHF is moderate.
d. The probability that her symptoms are related to CHF is high.
e. The probability that her symptoms are related to CHF is indeterminate.

166. You are seeing a sedentary, obese 41-year-old woman who presents to you with acute shortness of breath. She has tachycardia, but no other abnormal examination findings. You order a D-dimer and it comes back low. Which of the following is the most appropriate option?

a. Order a spiral CT of the chest.
b. Order a ventilation-perfusion (V̇/Q̇) scan.
c. Order Doppler flow studies of her lower extremities.
d. Order a pulmonary angiogram.
e. Reassure the patient that her symptoms are not concerning at this time.

167. One of your patients is dying of end-stage breast cancer. She is complaining of dyspnea. Which of the following treatment options would be most beneficial?

a. Bronchodilators
b. Steroids
c. Anxiolytics
d. Opioids
e. Pulmonary rehabilitation program

168. A 23-year-old sexually active woman visits a free clinic, reporting a sudden onset of dysuria that began 2 days ago. On further questioning, she also reports urinary frequency, some back pain, and a pink discoloration to her urine. She denies vaginal discharge or irritation, and has been afebrile. The clinic has no microscope or urine dip sticks available. Based on this history, what is her most likely diagnosis?

a. Acute bacterial cystitis
b. Urethritis
c. Pyelonephritis
d. Interstitial cystitis
e. Vulvovaginitis

169. You suspect acute cystitis in an otherwise healthy woman. Which of the following features decrease the likelihood of a urinary tract infection (UTI)?

a. Absence of fever
b. Absence of urgency
c. Absence of frequency
d. Absence of dysuria
e. Absence of vaginal discharge

170. An 18-year-old woman is seeing you for back pain, frequency, and dysuria. She has never had a UTI in the past, and though she recently became sexually active, she denies vaginal discharge or risk for sexually transmitted infection. In this setting, when would a urine culture be necessary?

a. If a urine dipstick were negative
b. If a urine dipstick was positive for leukocyte esterase only
c. If a urine dipstick was positive for leukocyte esterase and blood
d. If a microscopic evaluation of her centrifuged urine revealed more than 5 WBCs per high-powered field
e. If a microscopic evaluation of her centrifuged urine revealed significant bacteriuria

171. You are evaluating a 25-year-old woman who reports frequent UTIs since getting married last year. In the last 12 months, she has had five documented infections that have responded well to antibiotic therapy. She has tried voiding after intercourse, she discontinued her use of a diaphragm, and tried acidification of her urine using oral ascorbic acid, but none of those measures decreased the incidence of infections. At this point, which of the following would be an acceptable prophylactic measure?

a. An antibiotic prescription for the usual 3-day regimen with refills, to be used when symptoms occur
b. Single dose antibiotic therapy once daily at bedtime for 12 months
c. Single dose antibiotic therapy once daily at bedtime for 2 years
d. Single dose antibiotic therapy after sexual intercourse
e. Antibiotics for 3 days after sexual intercourse

172. A 36-year-old woman comes to your office complaining of recurrent dysuria. This is her fourth episode in the past 10 months. Initially, her symptoms were "classic" for a UTI. She was treated without obtaining urine dipstick or microscopic evaluation. For the second episode, her urinalysis was positive for blood only. Her culture was negative, as was evaluation for nephrolithiasis. The third episode was similar, also with a negative culture. All episodes have resolved with a standard course of antibiotic therapy. Which of the following is the most appropriate next step?

a. Evaluate for somatization disorder
b. Order cystoscopy
c. Treat for chronic vaginitis
d. Use a 14-day regimen of antibiotics
e. Use daily single-dose antibiotic therapy for prophylaxis

173. A screening urinalysis in a female patient reveals asymptomatic bacteriuria. In which of the following patients would treatment be indicated?

a. A sexually active teenager
b. A pregnant 26-year-old woman
c. A 45-year-old woman with uncontrolled hypertension
d. A menopausal woman
e. An otherwise healthy 80-year-old woman

174. You are seeing a 34-year-old man with urinary symptoms. He reports frequency, urgency, and moderate back pain. He is febrile and acutely ill. He has no penile discharge. His urinalysis shows marked pyuria. He has never had an episode like this before, and has no known urinary tract abnormalities. Which of the following is the most likely diagnosis?

a. Gonococcal urethritis
b. Nongonococcal urethritis
c. Acute bacterial cystitis
d. Pyelonephritis
e. Acute prostatitis

175. You care for a Caucasian family with five children. The 3-year-old is complaining of ear pain. He has a heart murmur and a family history of severe seasonal allergies. He has not been immunized. Of the things described which is considered to be a risk factor for acute otitis media?

a. Caucasian
b. Size of his family
c. Heart murmur
d. Family history of allergies
e. No immunizations

176. You are seeing a 25-year-old patient complaining of a left-sided earache. She describes the pain as deep, and worse with eating. Her ear examination is normal, but she has tenderness and crepitus during palpation of the left temporomandibular joint. Which of the following would be the most appropriate next step?

a. Antibiotic therapy
b. Treatment with NSAIDs
c. Dental referral
d. MRI of the temporomandibular joint
e. Obtaining an ESR

177. The mother of a 9-month-old infant brings him in for irritability. The child has been fussy and has not been sleeping well for 2 days. His highest temperature has been 100°F, and he has had a clear runny nose and a cough. On examination, the child is crying and irritable. Which physical examination finding, by itself, is insufficient to diagnose acute otitis media?

a. Opaque tympanic membrane
b. Bulging tympanic membrane
c. Impaired tympanic membrane mobility
d. Erythematous tympanic membrane
e. Purulent discharge in the ear canal

178. You are seeing a 4-year-old male 2 weeks after being diagnosed with left acute otitis media. He completed his therapy, is afebrile, acting well, and apparently back to normal. On examination, he has a persistent effusion in the left ear. There is no erythema, purulence, or hearing loss. Which of the following is the most appropriate next step?

a. Reassurance and reevaluation in 2 to 4 weeks
b. Ten-day course of a second-line antibiotic
c. Regular use of a decongestant and reevaluation in 2 weeks
d. Regular use of an antihistamine and reevaluation in 2 weeks
e. Referral to an otolaryngologist

179. You are seeing a 6-year-old patient whose mother brought him in for ear pain and fever. On examination, he is febrile, and his right tympanic membrane is shown below:

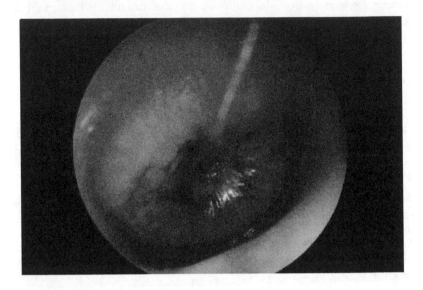

Which of the following would be the best initial treatment?

a. A weight-adjusted dose of Tylenol
b. A weight-adjusted course of amoxicillin
c. A weight-adjusted one-time dose of azithromycin
d. A weight-adjusted 3-day course of azithromycin
e. A weight-adjusted 5-day course of azithromycin

180. You are seeing a 16-year-old student complaining of ear pain. His pain has been present for 2 days. He denies fever and has no symptoms of upper respiratory infection. On examination, his ear canal is tender, erythematous, and swollen. His tympanic membrane is obscured by discharge and debris. Which of the following is the treatment of choice for this patient?

a. Flushing of the ear canal with hydrogen peroxide
b. Acetic acid washes
c. Topical antibiotics
d. Systemic antibiotics
e. Oral steroids

181. You are seeing a 45-year-old diabetic woman who reports bilateral lower extremity peripheral edema. In addition to diabetes, she has hypertension and depression. Which of the following medications is the likely cause of her edema?

a. Fluoxetine
b. Metformin
c. Rosiglitazone
d. Lisinopril
e. Hydrochlorothiazide

182. You are evaluating a 47-year-old woman complaining of bilateral lower extremity edema. She denies dyspnea, and on examination has no rales, JVD, or ascites. Her cardiac examination is normal. What should be the next step in the evaluation of her edema?

a. Echocardiogram
b. Thyroid-stimulating hormone (TSH) assessment
c. Liver function studies
d. Lower extremity Doppler
e. Urinalysis

183. You are evaluating a 40-year-old woman with a new onset of bilateral lower extremity edema. She denies dyspnea, and on examination has no rales or JVD. On evaluation, she has an abdominal fluid wave. Which of the following should be the next step in the evaluation of her edema?

a. Echocardiogram
b. TSH assessment
c. Liver function tests
d. Lower extremity Doppler
e. Urinalysis

184. You are evaluating a 38-year-old man complaining of swelling of his right leg. He denies dyspnea. On examination, he is obese. You note pitting edema on the right without signs of trauma, erythema, or inflammation. Which of the following would be the most appropriate next step in the evaluation of his edema?

a. Echocardiogram
b. Lower extremity Doppler
c. Spiral CT scan of his lungs
d. V/Q scan
e. Urinalysis

185. You are evaluating a 63-year-old diabetic man who noted unilateral lower extremity edema. He denies dyspnea or recent trauma. On evaluation, you note pitting edema on the right with well-demarcated erythema from the ankle to the mid thigh. Which of the following is the most likely diagnosis?

a. Varicose veins
b. Chronic CHF
c. Venous insufficiency
d. Deep venous thrombosis (DVT)
e. Cellulitis

186. You are evaluating a 55-year-old man with hypertension and hyper-lipidemia who complains of unilateral lower extremity edema. It has been present on and off for almost a year. He denies dyspnea or recent trauma, and has no evidence of inflammation. Which of the following would the best treatment option for his condition?

a. Diuresis
b. Anticoagulants
c. Elastic stockings
d. Sodium restriction
e. Angiotensin-converting enzyme (ACE) inhibitor

187. You are evaluating a 5-year-old girl brought in by her parents to discuss enuresis. She was toilet trained in the daytime at the age of 3 years, and was dry at night at about 3½ years of age. Four months ago, her parents had another child, and the 5-year-old began to wet the bed at night. She has no medical condition that would account for the change. Which of the following terms correctly describes this condition?

a. Primary nocturnal enuresis
b. Primary diurnal enuresis
c. Secondary nocturnal enuresis
d. Secondary diurnal enuresis
e. Primary intentional enuresis

188. You are seeing a 6-year-old girl whose parents brought her in to have her bed-wetting evaluated. She has been toilet trained during the day since the age of 4, but still wets the bed at night. Her father wet the bed until the age of 8 years. Her physical examination reveals no abnormalities, and her urinalysis is normal. Which of the following statements is true regarding this situation?

a. Up to 20% of 6-year-olds are enuretic.
b. Her father's history is inconsequential in this situation.
c. It is unusual for young girls to have a problem with enuresis.
d. The problem is likely due to her being a deep sleeper than other children.
e. There is likely an organic cause to her problem.

189. You are counseling a parent whose 7-year-old son wets the bed at night. Which of the following interventions has proven to be the most effective for this condition?

a. Frequent nighttime wakening to encourage voiding
b. Use of an alarm that wakes the child when he wets at night
c. Use of desmopressin (synthetic DDAVP)
d. Use of tricyclic antidepressant medications (eg, imipramine)
e. Use of an anticholinergic antispasmodic (eg, oxybutynin)

190. You are evaluating a 6-year-old boy. His mother has brought him in because he wets the bed. He has never been dry at night, and his parents are starting to get concerned. You obtain a thorough voiding history, and find the child to be completely normal on physical examination. He is otherwise developmentally normal. His urinalysis is also normal. What should be the next step in the workup of this patient?

a. Observation
b. X-rays of the lumbar and sacral spine
c. Renal ultrasound
d. Voiding cystourethrogram (VCUG)
e. Both renal ultrasound and VUCG

191. One of the children in your practice is troubled by nocturnal enuresis. He is 7 years old, and has avoided overnight activities with friends. Which of the following is the best initial treatment measure?

a. Treatment of constipation
b. Motivational therapy with consequences for not maintaining a dry bed
c. Desmopressin acetate (DDAVP)
d. Imipramine (Tofranil)
e. Tolterodine (Detrol)

192. You are discussing enuresis therapy with the mother of an 8-year-old girl that you care for. She is not interested in pharmacologic therapies, but would like to discuss using a moisture-sensitive alarm. Which of the following is true regarding the use of these alarms for nocturnal enuresis?

a.   The goal of this alarm is to wake the child just after the initiation of urination.
b.   The success rate is greater for boys than for girls.
c.   The success rate is less than 50%.
d.   If the process will be successful, it only takes 3 to 4 weeks on average.
e.   The alarms are easier for families because the child takes responsibility for the treatment.

193. You are seeing a 13-month-old Caucasian boy. His growth chart is shown. His past medical history and physical examination are otherwise unremarkable, and he is meeting his developmental milestones. Which of the following is most likely to reveal the cause of his growth pattern?

a.   Thorough dietary history
b.   Serum albumin levels
c.   Serum prealbumin levels
d.   Assessment of the TSH
e.   Serum IgA levels

Birth to 36 months: Boys
Length-for-age and Weight-for-age percentiles

NAME _____

RECORD # _____

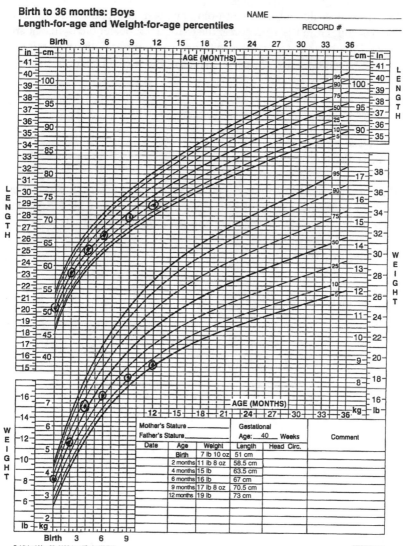

Date	Age	Weight	Length	Head Circ.
	Birth	7 lb 10 oz	51 cm	
	2 months	11 lb 8 oz	58.5 cm	
	4 months	15 lb	63.5 cm	
	6 months	16 lb	67 cm	
	9 months	17 lb 8 oz	70.5 cm	
	12 months	19 lb	73 cm	

Mother's Stature _____
Father's Stature _____
Gestational Age: __40__ Weeks
Comment

Published May 30, 2000 (modified 4/20/01).
SOURCE: Developed by the National Center for Health Statistics in collaboration with
the National Center for Chronic Disease Prevention and Health Promotion (2000).
http://www.cdc.gov/growthcharts

SAFER · HEALTHIER · PEOPLE™

194. You are evaluating a 9-month-old Caucasian girl for poor weight gain. She has gone from the 75th percentile to the 10th percentile in height and weight. She has had recurrent respiratory infections and diarrhea, but cultures obtained have been negative. Which of the following will be the most useful test in this setting?

a. Mantoux test for tuberculosis
b. Assessment for human immunodeficiency virus (HIV)
c. Stool for ova and parasites
d. Sweat chloride test
e. Renal function tests

195. You are seeing a 15-month-old boy for a well-child check. His parents have no concerns and his developmental history is normal. His growth chart is shown. Which of the following is the most likely observation?

a. Familial short stature
b. Failure to thrive
c. Hypothyroidism
d. A normal breast-fed infant
e. Constitutional growth delay

Birth to 36 months: Boys
Length-for-age and Weight-for-age percentiles

NAME _

RECORD # _____

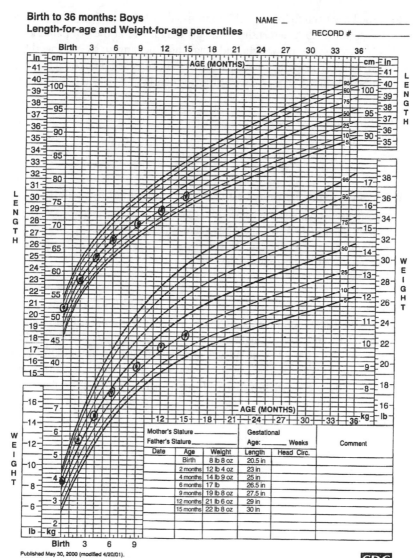

Date	Age	Weight	Length	Head Circ.
	Birth	8 lb 8 oz	20.5 in	
	2 months	12 lb 4 oz	23 in	
	4 months	14 lb 9 oz	25 in	
	6 months	17 lb	26.5 in	
	9 months	19 lb 8 oz	27.5 in	
	12 months	21 lb 6 oz	29 in	
	15 months	22 lb 8 oz	30 in	

Mother's Stature _____
Father's Stature _____
Gestational Age: _____ Weeks
Comment

Published May 30, 2000 (modified 4/20/01).
SOURCE: Developed by the National Center for Health Statistics in collaboration with
the National Center for Chronic Disease Prevention and Health Promotion (2000).
http://www.cdc.gov/growthcharts

SAFER·HEALTHIER·PEOPLE™

196. You have been following a 15-month-old male infant. At 9 months, his height was at the 25th percentile while his weight was at the 5th percentile. At his 12-month visit, his weight and height are unchanged, so you asked his family to bring in a detailed dietary history and counseled them on a healthy diet. At his 15-month visit, his weight is up slightly, and his vital signs are as follows:

Blood pressure:	62/32 mm Hg (low)
Heart rate:	72 beats per minute
Respiratory rate:	16 breaths per minute
Temperature:	98.8°F

Which of the following is the best therapeutic option for this child?

a. Nutritional instruction to take two times the normal caloric intake
b. Iron supplementation with increased calorie intake
c. Zinc with increased caloric intake
d. Referral to social services for neglect
e. Hospital admission

197. A 19-year-old male presented to your office with a 3-day history of fatigue, sore throat, and low-grade fevers. On examination, his temperature was 100.3°F, and you noted an exudative pharyngitis with cervical adenopathy. You sent a throat culture and started him on amoxicillin prophylactically. Two days later, he presents for follow up with continued symptoms and a diffuse, symmetrical erythematous maculopapular rash. Which of the following is the most likely cause of his symptoms?

a. Scarlet fever
b. Allergic reaction to amoxicillin
c. Viral exanthem
d. Mononucleosis
e. Measles

√ **198.** A 48-year-old man presents with a history of "feeling tired" for about 6 months. His previous doctor told him he probably had chronic fatigue syndrome, and he is presenting to you for a second opinion. He reports that his sleep is not refreshing. He has postexertional fatigue, weight loss, and also reports impaired concentration and headaches. Which of the following symptoms is less likely to be associated with chronic fatigue syndrome?

a. Unrefreshing sleep
b. Postexertional fatigue
c. Weight loss
d. Impaired concentration
e. Headaches

199. A 23-year-old woman presents to your office to discuss fatigue. She describes a "lack of energy" and "tiredness," but denies weakness or hypersomnolence. Which of the following is the next step in the workup?

a. Screen for depression
b. Screen for sleep apnea
c. Screen for anemia
d. Screen for hypothyroidism
e. Screen for pregnancy

√ **200.** You are discussing fatigue with one of your 53-year-old female patients. She reports that her symptoms have occurred for the past 6 months, and have been getting progressively worse. She reports increased stress and working longer hours at work, and she is drinking a glass of red wine each evening after work to relax. Which component of her history points to a physical cause of her fatigue?

a. Symptoms for 6 months
b. Progressively worsening
c. Associated with increased stress
d. Occurring when working longer hours
e. Alcohol overuse

201. You are evaluating a 56-year-old African American man complaining of fatigue. He describes this as a lack of stamina, but has motivation to do things. Sleep refreshes him, but he tires quickly at work. His physical examination is unremarkable. Which of the following should be included in your initial workup to help ascertain the diagnosis?

a. Chest x-ray
b. ECG
c. HIV test
d. Prostate cancer screen
e. Drug screen

202. A mother brings her son in to see you. He is almost 2 years old, and had a significant amount of painless bleeding from his rectum last evening. He is currently hemodynamically stable, and in no distress when you see him. Which of the following is the most likely diagnosis?

a. Juvenile polyposis
b. Colitis
c. Anal fissure
d. Intussusception
e. Meckel diverticulum

203. A 34-year-old man reports a 1-day history of hematemesis. He feels well, but does describe occasional abdominal discomfort. He denies alcohol use. On examination, his abdomen is slightly tender without peritoneal signs. His stool is not bloody, but his fecal test for occult blood is positive. Which of the following is the most appropriate next step?

a. Gastric lavage
b. Barium study
c. Endoscopy
d. Red cell scan
e. Angiography

204. You are evaluating a 44-year-old man with painless, large volume intestinal hemorrhage. You suspect a Meckel diverticulum as the possible cause. Which of the following is the best test to confirm this diagnosis?

a. Esophagogastroduodenoscopy
b. Sigmoidoscopy
c. Colonoscopy
d. Technetium-99m pertechnetate scintigraphic study
e. Laparotomy

205. A 56-year-old man is found to have asymptomatic diverticulosis on screening colonoscopy. He is concerned about his risk for GI bleeding from the diverticula. Which of the following statements is most accurate regarding his concern?

a. Severe diverticular bleeding is relatively common, occurring in up to 50% of patients with diverticulosis.
b. Diverticular bleeding is usually triggered by the ingestion of nuts, berries, seeds, popcorn, or other relatively indigestible material.
c. Diverticular bleeding resolves spontaneously in the vast majority of cases.
d. In patients with diverticular bleeding undergoing colonoscopy, blood emanating from a diverticulum is usually seen.
e. If colonoscopy fails to localize the source of active bleeding, a subtotal colectomy is needed to ensure no future bleeding.

206. You are evaluating a 26-year-old man with rectal pain. The pain was initially associated with bright red blood on the toilet paper after a bowel movement. Over the last day, his pain has worsened. On examination, he has an exquisitely tender purple nodule distal to the dentate line. Which of the following is the best treatment for his condition?

a. Hydrocortisone suppositories
b. Rubber band ligation
c. Sclerotherapy
d. Incision and drainage
e. Excision

207. You are evaluating a 30-year-old male patient in the office with hematochezia. He has had chronic constipation, and reports bright red blood from his rectum associated with extremely painful bowel movements. After defecation, he complains of a dull ache and a feeling of "spasm" in the anal canal. The pain resolves within a few hours. On external examination, no abnormalities are noted. Which of the following is his most likely diagnosis?

a. Anal fissure
b. Thrombosed external hemorrhoid
c. Internal hemorrhoid
d. Thrombosed internal hemorrhoid
e. Perianal abscess

208. You are evaluating a patient with a headache. Which of the following is most important in characterizing the type of headache the patient is experiencing?

a. History
b. Physical examination
c. Blood work
d. Imaging
e. Consultation with neurology

209. You are talking with a 24-year-old woman complaining of a headache. She reports that before she has the headache, she experiences visual symptoms associated with slight nausea. When the headache occurs later, it is throbbing, pulsating, and unilateral. During the headache, she experiences light sensitivity. Sleep improves the symptoms. Her symptoms are disrupting her daily life, and you decide to try prophylactic therapy. Which of the following is the most studied prophylactic agent to use?

a. β-Blockers
b. Calcium channel blockers
c. Selective serotonin reuptake inhibitors (SSRIs)
d. Anticonvulsants
e. Ergotamines

210. One of your patients has been on β-blocker therapy for migraine prophylaxis. Her symptoms are not controlled and she is interested in trying another prophylactic medication. Which class of antidepressants has the strongest evidence base for prophylactic use in migraines?

a. Tricyclic antidepressants
b. SSRIs
c. Monoamine oxidase inhibitors (MAOIs)
d. Selective norepinephrine reuptake inhibitors
e. Bupropion

211. You are caring for a patient who is complaining of a headache. Which of the following, if present, represents a "red flag" and necessitates a workup?

a. Headache that presents after the age of 50 years
b. Headache with a consistent location
c. Frequent, severe headaches
d. Visual disturbances with the headache
e. Severe nausea with the headache

212. You are seeing a 27-year-old male migraine sufferer. His attacks happen approximately monthly, and he would like to discuss abortive therapy. Which of the following options is rarely needed in the abortive treatment plan for migraine patients?

a. Acetaminophen
b. NSAIDs
c. Serotonin agonists
d. Ergotamines
e. Narcotics

213. You are discussing migraine management with a 30-year-old woman. She wants to use prophylactic medications, but had debilitating fatigue and symptoms of depression on β-blockers. Which of the following medications is an acceptable alternative?

a. Nifedipine
b. Verapamil
c. Diltiazem
d. Amlodipine
e. Nicardipine

214. A 38-year-old man comes to the office to discuss his headache symptoms. He describes the headaches as severe and intense, "like an ice pick in my eye!" The headaches begin suddenly, are unilateral, last up to 2 hours, and are associated with a runny nose and watery eye on the affected side. He gets several attacks over a couple of months, but is symptom-free for months in-between flare ups. Which of the following is the best approach for prophylactic management of the attacks?

a. SSRIs
b. Triptans
c. NSAIDs ·
d. Calcium channel blockers
e. Ergotamine

215. A 42-year-old man that you treat suffers from cluster headaches. He would like a medication to take when he has an attack (abortive therapy). Which of the following would be best for treatment of the acute episodes?

a. Indomethacin, 120 mg by mouth
b. Oxycodone, 5 to 10 mg by mouth
c. Sumatriptan, 50 to 100 mg by mouth
d. Ergotamine, 1 to 2 mg by mouth
e. Hundred percent oxygen, administered via a nasal canula

216. You are talking with a 33-year-old woman who is complaining of headaches. She has had these headaches for 5 months, and they are increasing in frequency. She reports that the headaches may last anywhere from an hour to several days. They are now occurring about 5 to 10 times a month, without relationship to her menstrual cycle. She describes the headache as bilateral, and the pain is described as a pressure around her forehead. She denies nausea, is not sensitive to sound, but is sensitive to light during an attack. On examination, she has no obvious neurological deficit. Which of the following is the best approach to take at this point?

a.   Prescribe narcotic analgesics and follow up if no improvement
b.   Prescribe NSAIDs and follow up if no improvement
c.   Order blood work to rule out secondary cause
d.   Order a CT of the brain
e.   Order an MRI of the brain

217. You are caring for a 54-year-old with a new complaint of headaches. They are described as unilateral and throbbing in nature, and began 2 months ago. There is associated photophobia and nausea. In this history, what feature is most concerning for a secondary headache?

a.   Unilateral
b.   Throbbing
c.   Recent onset
d.   Photophobia
e.   Nausea

218. You are taking care of a 32-year-old woman with mild hypertension, arthritis, and depression. She presents to you complaining of a sore throat without cough or congestion. You diagnose her with pharyngitis and begin treatment. She then has an acute onset of hematuria, and comes to your office for evaluation. Which of the following medications used to treat pharyngitis is the most likely cause?

a.   Ibuprofen
b.   Penicillin
c.   Azithromycin
d.   Erythromycin
e.   Ciprofloxacin

219. You are evaluating a 56-year-old generally healthy man who is seeing you after finding blood in his urine. He denies pain, dysuria, frequency, or urgency. He is a smoker, and has worked for years in the printing industry. Which of the following is the most likely cause of his hematuria?

a. Acute prostatitis
b. Chronic prostatitis
c. Cystitis
d. Urinary stones
e. Bladder carcinoma

220. A 16-year-old girl comes to your office complaining of blood in her urine. She is asymptomatic, and not menstruating. Urinalysis reveals grossly pink urine, but urine dipstick is negative for blood. Which of the following foods is the likely cause?

a. Spinach
b. Strawberries
c. Raspberries
d. Beets
e. Carrots

221. A 62-year-old man is seeing you because he noted blood in his urine. He states that the blood appears at the end of urination, and is not associated with other symptoms (pain, frequency, or urgency). Which of the following is the most likely cause of his hematuria?

a. Urethral cancer
b. Renal cancer
c. Prostate cancer
d. Urolithiasis
e. Urethral trauma

222. You are seeing a 14-year-old boy who reports seeing blood in his urine. He is currently asymptomatic. On urinalysis, he has more than 10 RBC per high-powered field, he has red cell casts, and his creatinine is 2.3 mg/dL (H). Which of the following is the next step in the evaluation?

a. IV pyelography
b. Renal ultrasound
c. Cystoscopy
d. Noncontrast helical CT
e. Antistreptolysin O (ASO) titer

223. On a routine urinalysis, a 30-year-old man was found to have hematuria. His urinalysis is negative for casts and protein, but is positive for moderate blood. His urine culture is negative. IV pyelogram and serum creatinine are both normal. Which of the following is most appropriate in this case?

a. Reassurance and periodic monitoring
b. Renal ultrasound
c. Cystoscopy
d. ASO titer
e. Renal biopsy

224. A day-care worker presents to your office after turning "yellow." She reports feeling feverish and fatigued, and describes right upper quadrant abdominal pain and nausea. On examination, her skin tone, conjunctivae, and mucous membranes are yellow-tinged. Serologies indicate acute hepatitis A infection. Which of the following is true about this infection?

a. She is most infectious while she is jaundiced.
b. Fecal shedding of the virus continues until liver enzymes have normalized.
c. Complete recovery is the norm.
d. Relapses are common.
e. This infection can lead to chronic infection.

225. A patient is seeing you in follow-up after being hospitalized for acute hepatitis. He is concerned about his risk for hepatocellular carcinoma. Which form of viral hepatitis is associated with a clearly increased risk of hepatocellular carcinoma?

a. Hepatitis A virus
b. Hepatitis B virus
c. Hepatitis C virus
d. Hepatitis D virus
e. Hepatitis E virus

✓ **226.** You are examining a newborn whose mother has a positive screen for hepatitis B surface antigen (HBsAg). Which of the following is true regarding this situation?

a. When acquired early in life, the large majority of those infected with hepatitis B will have chronic disease.
b. If the child has a normal immune system, his likelihood of developing chronic disease is small.
c. A higher percentage of adults infected with hepatitis B will develop chronic disease as compared with children.
d. A high percentage of children acutely infected will develop fulminant liver disease.
e. When hepatitis B is transmitted perinatally, the child generally develops the typical symptoms of acute hepatitis.

227. One of your patients had unprotected intercourse with a partner later found to have chronic hepatitis B. In testing your patient, which of the following serologic markers would be the first to appear?

a. Hepatitis B surface antigen (HBsAg)
b. Hepatitis B core antigen (HBcAg)
c. The IgM to the core protein (IgM anti-HBc)
d. Hepatitis B e antigen (HBeAg)
e. The IgM to HBeAg

228. You are talking with a patient who recently found out that a coworker has hepatitis C. Which of the following is true about hepatitis C?

a. The hepatitis C virus is found in blood
b. The hepatitis C virus is found in semen
c. The hepatitis C virus is found in vaginal secretions
d. The hepatitis C virus is found in breast milk
e. The hepatitis C virus is found in saliva

✓ **229.** You are following a patient after an acute hepatitis B infection. His serologies are shown below:

- HBsAg: Positive
- HBeAg: Positive
- IgM anti-HBc: Negative
- IgG anti-HBc: Positive
- Anti-HBs: Negative
- Anti-HBe: Negative
- HBV-DNA: Positive

Which of the following terms best describes his disease status?

a. Acute infection, early phase
b. Acute infection, recovery phase
c. Chronic infection, replicating virus
d. Chronic infection, nonreplicating virus
e. Previous exposure with immunity

230. You check serologies on a patient exposed to hepatitis B. His serologies are shown below:

- HBsAg: Negative
- HBeAg: Negative
- IgM anti-HBc: Negative
- IgG anti-HBc: Negative
- Anti-HBs: Positive
- Anti-HBe: Negative
- HBV-DNA: Negative

Which of the following terms best describes his disease status?

a. Acute infection, early phase
b. Acute infection, window phase
c. Acute infection, recovery phase
d. Previous exposure with immunity
e. Vaccination

231. You are following a patient after an acute hepatitis B infection. His serologies are shown below:

- HBsAg: Positive
- HBeAg: Positive
- IgM anti-HBc: Positive
- IgG anti-HBc: Negative
- Anti-HBs: Negative
- Anti-HBe: Negative
- HBV-DNA: Positive

Which of the following terms best describes his disease status?

a. Acute infection, early phase
b. Acute infection, recovery phase
c. Chronic infection, replicating virus.
d. Chronic infection, nonreplicating virus
e. Previous exposure with immunity

232. A 62-year-old woman describes mild loss of urine at times. Which of the following normal age-related phenomenon is true?

a. Overflow incontinence may occur because the frequency of involuntary bladder contractions decreases with age.
b. Urge incontinence may occur because total bladder capacity decreases with age.
c. Stress incontinence may occur because total bladder contractility increases with age.
d. Overflow incontinence may occur because elderly patients excrete a larger percentage of fluid earlier in the day.
e. Urge incontinence may occur because elderly women have urogenital atrophy due to decreased estrogen.

233. You are evaluating a 74-year-old woman for the recent onset of incontinence. She has diabetes, controlled by diet but with recently increasing sugars, and hypertension, controlled with a combination of lisinopril/ hydrochlorothiazide. She has complained of constipation recently, and has not had a bowel movement for 3 days. Microscopic analysis of her urine is positive for bacteria, but she does not report dysuria, urgency, or frequency. Which of the historical features mentioned is inconsequential in the workup of her incontinence?

a. Hyperglycemia
b. Diuretic use
c. Constipation
d. Bacteriuria
e. Postmenopausal state

234. You are caring for a 42-year-old woman complaining of incontinence. She reports often having a strong, often immediate need to void, followed by an involuntary loss of urine. She says her symptoms develop so suddenly, she often urinates while trying to get to the bathroom. Which of the following best describes the type of incontinence she is experiencing?

a. Functional incontinence
b. Senile incontinence
c. Urge incontinence
d. Stress incontinence
e. Overflow incontinence

235. A 44-year-old mother of two reports leakage of a small amount of urine with sneezing. Recently, it began to occur with exercise. She denies recent life stressors. Which of the following best describes the type of incontinence she is experiencing?

a. Functional incontinence
b. Senile incontinence
c. Urge incontinence
d. Stress incontinence
e. Overflow incontinence

236. One of your patients, a 70-year-old man, complains of frequently dribbling urine throughout the day. On occasion, he loses a large amount of urine without warning. He is otherwise healthy and takes no other medications. Based on his profile and symptoms, which of the following terms best describes his symptoms?

a. Functional incontinence
b. Senile incontinence
c. Urge incontinence
d. Stress incontinence
e. Overflow incontinence

237. You are seeing a 74-year-old man who is complaining that he is leaking urine. You have ruled out secondary causes, and choose to measure his "postvoid" residual. It is 250 mL. Which of the following is true?

a. Postvoid residual measurement has no place in the workup of incontinence.
b. This amount is below what is expected, and leads one to suspect urge incontinence.
c. This amount is about average, and is not helpful in determining this patient's type of incontinence.
d. This amount is more than average, but is not helpful in determining this patient's type of incontinence.
e. This amount is more than average, and would lead one to suspect overflow incontinence.

238. You are treating a 40-year-old woman for incontinence. She'd prefer not to use medications, and would like to try pelvic floor strengthening (Kegel) exercises. Which of the following types of incontinence has shown the best response to pelvic floor strengthening exercises?

a. Functional incontinence
b. Stress incontinence
c. Urge incontinence
d. Overflow incontinence
e. Mixed incontinence

239. One of your patients has tried and failed behavioral therapy for incontinence. He describes a strong urge to urinate, followed by involuntary loss of urine. Which of the following would be the best medication for him to use?

a. Oxybutynin (Ditropan)
b. Pseudoephedrine (Sudafed)
c. Trimethoprim-sulfamethoxazole (Bactrim, Septra)
d. Finasteride (Proscar)
e. Terazosin (Hytrin)

240. You are treating a 45-year-old man for hypertension. Since beginning therapy, he complains of urinary leakage and urgency. Which antihypertensive class is most likely to cause this?

a. Thiazide diuretics
b. ACE inhibitors
c. β-Blockers
d. Calcium channel blockers
c. α-Blockers

241. An obese 29-year-old woman is complaining of polyuria. Her workup, including serum glucose, is negative. She is not taking any prescription medications. Which of the following, if present in her history, is the most likely cause?

a. Marijuana abuse
b. Over-the-counter diet pill use
c. Over-the-counter decongestant use
d. Over-the-counter sleeping pill use
e. Caffeine over-use

242. You are evaluating a 14-year-old female patient whose mother brought her in for evaluation. Despite the fact that all of her friends have started menstruating, the daughter has not. On examination, she has no breast development, no axillary or pubic hair, and her pelvic examination reveals normal-appearing anatomy. She has not lost weight recently and is not excessively thin. Which of the following is the most likely cause of her primary amenorrhea?

a. Gonadal dysgenesis
b. Hypothalamic failure
c. Pituitary failure
d. Polycystic ovarian syndrome
e. Constitutional delay of puberty

243. You are seeing a 17-year-old patient who began menstruating at age 14, and has been relatively regular since age 15. She made an appointment to be seen today because she stopped having periods 2 months ago. She denies sexual activity. Which of the following is the most common cause of secondary amenorrhea?

a. Polycystic ovarian syndrome
b. Functional hypothalamic amenorrhea
c. Pregnancy
d. Hypothyroidism
e. Hyperprolactinemia

√**244.** A 16-year-old woman comes to your office complaining of unpredictable menstrual periods. She began her periods at age 14, and they have never been predictable. She denies sexual activity in her lifetime, has no systemic illness, uses no medications regularly, and her physical examination is normal. Which of the following is her most likely diagnosis?

a. Pregnancy
b. Ovulatory bleeding
c. Anovulatory bleeding
d. Uterine leiomyoma
e. Endometrial polyposis

√ **245.** A healthy 60-year-old woman is seeing you to evaluate vaginal bleeding. She has not had a menstrual period for approximately 7 years, but 3 months ago noted occasional pink spotting. Since then, it has increased in amount and has become almost continuous. She is currently sexually active with her husband. On examination, she appears well, her pelvic examination is normal, and screens for sexually transmitted infections are negative. Which of the following should be your next step?

a. Pelvic ultrasound to evaluate for fibroids
b. Pelvic CT scan to evaluate for pelvic tumor
c. Laparoscopy to evaluate for endometriosis
d. Endometrial biopsy
e. Begin hormone-replacement therapy to regulate bleeding

√**246.** You are considering treatment for a 19-year-old female patient with primary dysmenorrhea. Which of the following should be your first-line therapy?

a. Use of NSAIDs during menses
b. Use of NSAIDs daily
c. Use of opiates during menses
d. Use of an SSRI daily
e. Use of combined oral contraceptive pills daily

247. You are evaluating a 16-year-old who has not menstruated yet. She appears short in stature. Which of the following is the most likely genetic diagnosis?

a. Turner syndrome
b. Fragile X syndrome
c. Down syndrome
d. Testicular feminization syndrome
e. Factor V Leiden deficiency

√ **248.** You are evaluating a 32-year-old woman complaining of amenorrhea. She has mild hypertension, hypothyroidism, GERD, and depression. On evaluation, her prolactin level was found to be 89 ng/mL (H). Which of the following medications would be most likely to cause the elevated prolactin level?

a. Proton pump inhibitors
b. SSRIs
c. Thiazide diuretics
d. ACE inhibitors
e. Thyroid hormone replacement

249. You are evaluating 34-year-old woman reports amenorrhea for 4 months. She has never been "regular," but has never gone this long without a period. Her laboratory evaluation is normal, including a negative pregnancy test. You give her medroxyprogesterone acetate (Provera) for 7 days, and the next week, she reports having a period. Which of the following is the most likely cause of her amenorrhea?

a. Premature ovarian failure
b. Ovarian neoplasm
c. Turner syndrome
d. Asherman syndrome
e. Polycystic ovarian syndrome

250. A 45-year-old woman in your practice is complaining of amenorrhea. During the workup, you discover her testosterone and dehydroepiandros-terone sulphate (DHEA-S) levels are elevated. Which of the following should be your next step?

a. CT scanning of the adrenal glands
b. Hysteroscopy
c. Hysterosalpingogram
d. MRI of the brain
e. Karyotyping

251. You are evaluating a 16-year-old girl who has never menstruated. She has normal secondary sexual characteristics, and her laboratory evaluation is negative. She has no withdrawal bleeding after a progestin challenge, and you choose to perform an estrogen-progestin challenge. She has no withdrawal bleeding after that challenge as well. Which of the following is the most likely reason for her amenorrhea?

a. Outflow tract obstruction
b. Hypergonadotropic amenorrhea
c. Hypogonadotropic amenorrhea
d. Polycystic ovarian syndrome
e. Pituitary adenoma

✓ **252.** You are seeing a 24-year-old woman complaining of dysmenorrhea. She has always had painful periods, but lately they seem to be worsening. Her physical examination, including pelvic examination, is normal. She is not currently sexually active. Which of the following is the most appropriate next step in the workup?

a. No further workup is needed
b. Gonorrhea and *Chlamydia* cultures
c. Pelvic ultrasound
d. Hysterosalpingography
e. Laparoscopy

253. You are evaluating an 18-year-old college student complaining of painful menstrual periods. She reports that she began menstruating at age 14. Since that time, her periods have always been associated with pain. The pain begins just prior to her period starting, and lasts for up to 3 days. She has associated nausea, fatigue, and headache. Her history and physical examination are normal, and you choose to treat her with a trial of oral contraceptives. Which of the following describes how oral contraceptives work to treat dysmenorrhea?

a. Suppression of prostaglandin synthesis
b. Suppression of prostaglandin release
c. Induction of endometrial hyperplasia
d. Increase in vasoconstriction of the uterus
e. Direct decrease of uterine resting tone

254. You are caring for a 70-year-old hospitalized male who is currently 1 day out from a carotid endarterectomy. You are called to the floor at 3:00 AM because the patient removed his peripheral IV and is demanding to go home. Reviewing his chart, you see he has a history of hypertension and hyperlipidemia, both of which are well controlled with medication. He is working part time as an auto mechanic, and lives at home with his wife. On evaluation, he is agitated but responds to questions, is oriented to person only, and denies chest pain, palpitations, shortness of breath, dizziness, or other problems. Which of the following characteristics points to delirium instead of dementia in this case?

a. The acute onset of his symptoms
b. The fact that he is disoriented to time and place
c. His history of hypertension
d. The fact that he is responsive to questions
e. The fact that this happened in the early morning hours

255. You are in the emergency room caring for a 47-year-old man who was brought in by his wife. She states that he had the acute onset of confusion. His past medical history is unremarkable, without evidence of drug or alcohol use. On examination, you find his blood pressure to be 210/130 mm Hg, his pulse to be 97 beats per minute, and his respirations to be 20 breaths per minute. His temperature is 98.4°F. Strength, sensation, and gait are normal. He has no tremor. Which of the following would you expect to find on ophthalmologic examination?

a. Pinpoint pupils
b. Dilated pupils
c. Papilledema
d. Sixth cranial nerve palsy
e. Anisocoria of 1 mm

256. You are evaluating a homeless person in the emergency department who is displaying hyperalert confusion. Withdrawal from which of the following substances is most likely to cause this state?

a. Levothyroxine
b. Fluoxetine
c. Oxycodone/acetaminophen
d. Alcohol
e. Amphetamine

✓ **257.** You receive a telephone call from the mother of a 19-year-old patient. During the day, she complained of a headache, body aches, and a low-grade fever. She went to bed 30 minutes ago, and her mother is now finding it difficult to arouse her. Which of the following tests would be most likely to reveal the diagnosis?

a. Urinalysis
b. CBC
c. Toxicology screen
d. Pregnancy test
e. Lumbar puncture

✓ **258.** You are seeing a 78-year-old man who was brought to the office by his daughter. The daughter says her father is becoming increasingly forgetful. His medical history is significant for a 20-year history of type 2 diabetes and well-controlled hypertension. On examination, he is mildly hypertensive with otherwise normal vital signs. He is oriented to time, place, and person, but is unable to complete "serial sevens" on a mini-mental status examination. Which of the historical features make this diagnosis more consistent with dementia as opposed to delirium?

a. His history of hypertension
b. His history of diabetes
c. His current level of orientation
d. His inability to complete serial sevens
e. The recent onset of his symptoms

✓ **259.** A 53-year-old woman is seeing you because of chronic nausea and vomiting. She has a 15-year history of type 2 diabetes mellitus. Her symptoms are worse after eating, and on occasion she will vomit food that appears to be undigested. Her weight is stable and she does not appear dehydrated. Which of the following is the best treatment for her condition?

a. An anticholinergic medication, like scopolamine (Transderm Scop)
b. An antihistamine, like promethazine (Phenergan)
c. A benzamide, like metoclopramide (Reglan)
d. A cannabinoid, like dronabinol (Marinol)
e. A phenothiazine, like chlorpromazine (Thorazine)

260. You are evaluating a 63-year-old man who complains of abdominal pain, distension, nausea, and vomiting. It began rather suddenly this morning, though he has had mild pain for several days. His past history is significant for a partial sigmoid resection for diverticulosis and an appendectomy at 23 years of age. On examination, he is afebrile, his mucous membranes are dry, but he has no orthostatic symptoms. His abdomen is distended and diffusely tender, and his bowel sounds are hyperactive. Which of the following is the most likely cause of his nausea and vomiting?

a. Gastroenteritis
b. Ileus
c. Obstruction
d. Diverticulosis
e. Diverticulitis

261. You are seeing a 12-year-old girl for nausea and vomiting. She was diagnosed as having viral gastroenteritis in the emergency department more than 6 weeks ago, but since that time has had difficulty keeping food down. She states that whenever she eats, she gets nauseated and vomits within 10 to 30 minutes. She has been using antiemetics to control her symptoms, but they do not work consistently. She has always done well in school, and denies social stressors. Her medical history is unremarkable, but she was treated for depression last year. On examination, she is well-nourished, interactive, and in no distress with no signs of dehydration. Her weight is 147 lb (5 lb less than at her well examination 6 months ago) and her height is 5 ft. Which of the following is the most likely cause of her symptoms?

a. Chronic gastroenteritis
b. Psychogenic vomiting
c. Anorexia nervosa
d. Bulimia nervosa
e. Central nervous system malignancy

262. You are seeing a 6-year-old boy with nausea and vomiting. His symptoms began acutely last evening, starting with malaise, headache, low-grade fever, body aches, and diarrhea. On examination, he has dry mucous membranes, but no orthostatic symptoms. He has diffuse mild abdominal pain without rebound or involuntary guarding. Which of the following is the best treatment for his condition?

a. Nothing by mouth until his symptoms improve
b. Oral rehydration with clear liquids, advancing the diet as tolerated
c. IV rehydration, advancing to oral as tolerated
d. Antiemetics, given intravenously or intramuscularly
e. Trimethoprim/sulfamethoxazole therapy

263. You are seeing a 44-year-old woman with hypertension controlled with lisinopril, who presents with severe nausea and vomiting. She reports having months of occasional right upper quadrant pain, usually after eating out with her husband, that resolves within a couple of hours. Over the last 24 hours, her symptoms have been severe, and she is unable to eat or drink without vomiting. Her pain is significant, radiates to her back, and is better when she leans forward. On laboratory evaluation, her amylase is elevated, and her ALT is elevated. Which of the following would be the best approach to avoid recurrent problems in her case?

a. Discontinue lisinopril
b. Avoid calcium in the diet
c. Work with the patient to remain sober
d. Remove the patient's gallbladder
e. Use medication to lower the patient's triglyceride level

264. You are seeing a 48-year-old man who complains of nausea and vomiting. He is nauseated before breakfast, and he describes the vomiting as "severe" and "projectile." His symptoms are associated with headache and dizziness, but improve throughout the day. Which of the following is the most likely diagnosis?

a. Gastroparesis
b. Cholelithiasis
c. Pancreatitis
d. Vestibular disorder
e. Brain tumor

265. You are evaluating a 54-year-old obese woman who is complaining of nausea. She has not been to a doctor for more than 10 years. Her symptoms occur an hour or two after eating meals, and she denies any pain. Which of the following is the most likely diagnosis?

a. Gastroparesis
b. Cholelithiasis
c. Pancreatitis
d. Vestibular disorder
e. Brain tumor

266. A new mother brings her infant to see you to discuss his vomiting. He is 4 weeks old, and is exclusively breast-fed. He vomits with every meal. On examination, his abdomen is distended with normal bowel sounds, and he appears dehydrated. He has lost 4 oz since his visit with you 2 weeks ago. Which of the following is the most likely diagnosis?

a. Allergy to breast milk
b. GERD
c. Pyloric stenosis
d. Intussusception
e. Small-bowel obstruction

267. You are evaluating a 31-year-old man with the acute onset of nausea and vomiting. It is associated with significant epigastric pain that radiates to the back and occurs after eating any type of food. It is somewhat better if he does not eat at all. Which of the following tests is most likely to be abnormal in this case?

a. CBC
b. Amylase and lipase level assessment
c. Hemoccult testing of the stool
d. Abdominal x-rays
e. Upper endoscopy

268. A 42-year-old woman is seeing you to evaluate nausea and vomiting. It happens about 60 minutes after eating a big meal, and is associated with pain in the epigastric area. Which of the following tests is most likely to be abnormal in this case?

a. Amylase and lipase level assessment
b. Hemoccult testing of the stool
c. Abdominal x-rays
d. Ultrasound
e. Upper endoscopy

✓ **269.** You are treating a 26-year-old woman for nausea. Which of the following antiemetics is most likely to cause extrapyramidal reactions in the patient?

a. Trimethobenzamide (Tigan)
b. Prochlorperazine (Compazine)
c. Promethazine (Phenergan)
d. Metoclopramide (Reglan)
e. Ondansetron (Zofran)

270. You are evaluating a 33-year-old woman complaining of palpitations. Which of the following characteristics, if present, increase the likelihood that the symptoms are cardiac in etiology?

a. The fact that the patient is female
b. The fact that the patient has a sister with similar symptoms
c. Her description of the symptoms as an "irregular heartbeat"
d. The fact that her father has a history of heart disease
e. The fact that the episodes last less than 1 minute

271. You are seeing a hypertensive 56-year-old woman who is complaining of a "fluttering in her chest." She describes a rapid heart rate, and to her it seems irregular. She is otherwise well, and denies shortness of breath, light-headedness pedal edema, or other acute symptoms. On examination, her pulse rate is rapid and irregular. Which of the following is her most likely diagnosis?

a. Atrial fibrillation
b. Paroxysmal supraventricular tachycardia (PSVT)
c. Stable ventricular tachycardia
d. Stimulant abuse
e. Hyperthyroidism

272. You are seeing a 32-year-old otherwise healthy woman who is complaining of palpitations. She describes the sensation as a "flip flop" in her chest. They only last an instant, and are not associated with lightheadedness or other symptoms. She denies other symptoms. Which of the following is the most likely etiology of her complaint?

a. Atrial fibrillation
b. PSVT
c. Ventricular premature beats
d. Stimulant abuse
e. Hyperthyroidism

273. You are seeing a 19-year-old African American student who reports that he can "feel his heartbeat." It happens with exercise and is associated with some lightheadedness and shortness of breath. On examination, his heart has a regular rate and rhythm, but you hear a holosystolic murmur along his left sternal border. It increases with Valsalva maneuver. Which of the following is the most likely cause of his symptoms?

a. Mitral valve prolapse
b. Hypertrophic obstructive cardiomyopathy
c. Dilated cardiomyopathy
d. Atrial fibrillation
e. CHF

274. A 32-year-old woman reports that she sometimes "skips heartbeats." Her medical and social histories include moderate daily caffeine use, but are otherwise unremarkable. Her physical examination and 12-lead ECG are normal, as are her CBC, electrolytes, and TSH. Which of the following is the next appropriate step in her workup?

a. Reassure her and continue observation
b. Perform ambulatory ECG monitoring (a 24-Holter monitor, or a continuous loop event recorder)
c. Electrophysiology consultation
d. Stress testing
e. Echocardiography

275. You are evaluating a 23-year-old African American swimmer who is complaining of episodes of symptomatic rapid heart beating. Twice during swim practice, he develops a sensation that his heart is racing. When he measures his heart rate, he finds it to be between 140 to 160 beats per minute. The first episode lasted approximately 4 minutes, and the second lasted more than 10 minutes. He denies lightheadedness or other symptoms during the events. Limited laboratory evaluation and ECG are normal. Which of the following is the next step in the evaluation?

a. Reassure and continue observation
b. Ambulatory ECG monitoring
c. Consultation with an electrophysiologist
d. Stress testing
e. Echocardiography

276. You are seeing a man complaining of symptomatic palpitations. His ECG is shown below:

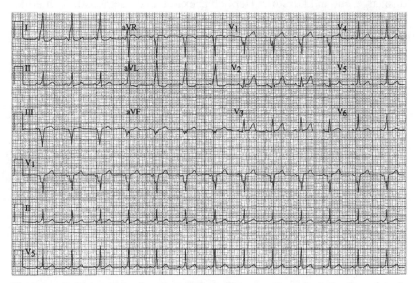

(Reproduced, with permission, from Ferry D. Basic Electrocardiography in Ten Days, 1st ed. New York: McGraw-Hill, 2001: 177.)

Which of the following is the likely diagnosis?

a. Sinus tachycardia
b. Supraventricular tachycardia
c. Wolff-Parkinson-White syndrome
d. Ventricular tachycardia
e. Premature atrial contractions

277. You are caring for a 23-year-old woman complaining of pelvic pain. She reports one-sided pain that is diffuse and dull, but occasionally sharp. Menses have been normal. She denies fever. Her pelvic examination is normal with the exception of a smooth mobile adnexal mass on the right side. Which of the following is the most likely cause of the pain?

a. Pelvic inflammatory disease (PID)
b. Ectopic pregnancy
c. Ovarian cyst
d. Uterine leiomyoma
e. Appendicitis

278. You are caring for a 21-year-old woman complaining of pelvic pain. She reports a gradual onset of bilateral pain associated with fever, vaginal discharge, and mild dysuria. Her pelvic examination demonstrates uterine, adnexal, and cervical motion tenderness. Which of the following is the most likely cause of the pain?

a. PID
b. Ectopic pregnancy
c. Ovarian cyst
d. Uterine leiomyoma
e. Appendicitis

279. You are caring for a 27-year-old woman complaining of pelvic pain. She reports localized pain on the left side that has increased in severity over the last 2 days. She also reports amenorrhea and nausea. On examination, you note a tender adnexal mass on the left. Which of the following is the most likely cause?

a. PID
b. Ectopic pregnancy
c. Ovarian cyst
d. Uterine leiomyoma
e. Appendicitis

280. You are evaluating a 33-year-old woman with chronic pelvic pain. She reports cyclic pain, generally during the premenstrual period and during her menses. She has been trying to conceive for 15 months without success. Her pelvic examination is normal. Which of the following tests would be most helpful in determining the cause of her pain?

a. CBC
b. ESR
c. CA-125 levels
d. Transvaginal pelvic ultrasound
e. MRI

✓ **281.** You are evaluating a 14-year-old girl with pelvic pain. She denies being sexually active and you do not suspect abuse. On pelvic examination, you confirm that she has never been sexually active, see no discharge and find no cervical motion tenderness, but feel an ovarian mass on the right side. Which of the following is the most appropriate next step in this situation?

a. Reassurance and use of NSAIDs for pain control
b. Reassurance and repeat pelvic examination in 6 to 8 weeks
c. Transvaginal pelvic ultrasound
d. CT scanning of the abdomen and pelvis
e. MRI evaluation of the pelvis

✓ **282.** You are evaluating an 18-year-old male with a sore throat. It has been present for 3 days, and is associated with fever, aches, and fatigue. On examination, he has an exudative pharyngitis, soft palate petechiae, and posterior cervical adenopathy. Which of the following is the most likely diagnosis?

a. Group A streptococcal infection
b. Group A streptococcal colonization
c. Corynebacterium diphtheriae infection
d. Gonorrhea infection of the throat
e. Epstein-Barr virus (EBV) infection

✓ **283.** A 7-year-old boy comes to see you for a sore throat. He reports fevers, chills, myalgias, and pain on swallowing. On examination, you note anterior adenopathy, erythematous tonsils, and edema of his uvula. He has no drug allergies. Which of the following would be the best treatment for his condition?

a. Symptomatic care
b. Antiviral therapy
c. Doxycycline (Vibramycin)
d. Amoxicillin (Amoxil)
e. Erythromycin (Emycin)

284. You are treating a 16-year-old girl with a sore throat. She denies runny nose or cough, but does report fevers and myalgia. On examination, she has an exudative pharyngitis, and posterior cervical adenopathy. Her rapid streptococcal antigen is positive. You treat her with penicillin, and she develops a diffuse maculopapular rash. Which of the following is the most likely diagnosis?

a. Scarlet fever
b. Infectious mononucleosis
c. Viral exanthem
d. Allergy to penicillin
e. Tinea versicolor

285. An 8-year-old patient has a history of testing positive for group A streptococcal throat infections whether or not he is symptomatic. You have determined that he is a streptococcal carrier. Assuming that the patient has no allergies, what is the best therapeutic option in this patient?

a. Penicillin (PenVK)
b. Amoxicillin (Amoxil), using the usual dose
c. Amoxicillin (Amoxil), using high dosages
d. Erythromycin (Emycin)
e. Clindamycin (Cleocin)

286. You are treating a 16-year-old patient with a sore throat. She has had 3 days of symptoms, and does not have nasal congestion or cough. She also reports laryngitis. On examination, she has an erythematous pharynx without exudate. Which of the following is the most appropriate therapy based on the symptoms described?

a. Supportive care
b. Penicillin (PenVK)
c. Amoxicillin (Amoxil)
d. Erythromycin (Emycin)
e. Clindamycin (Cleocin)

√ **287.** You are caring for a 9-year-old whose mother brought him in for evaluation of his sore throat. He has been ill for 24 hours. In addition to the sore throat, he has a fever, but no cough. On physical examination, his temperature is 101°F, tender anterior cervical adenopathy and tonsillar exudate. Which of the following is the next best step in his care?

a. Reassurance and observation for a few more days
b. Perform a rapid streptococcal screening test
c. Perform a throat culture
d. Treat with penicillin
e. Treat with steroids

√ **288.** You are caring for a teen with fairly severe acne. Which of the following has been shown to play a role in the development of acne?

a. Stress
b. Dirty skin
c. Chocolate
d. Increased greasy foods in the diet
e. Oily hair on the forehead

289. One of your patients is concerned about facial acne. He has both inflammatory and comedonal acne (see picture below), and you would rate it as moderate in severity. Which of the following would be the best approach to treating his acne?

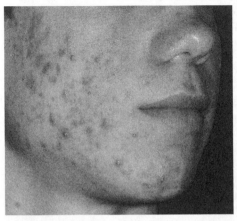

(Reproduced, with permission, from Wolff K, Johnson RA, Suurmond D. Fitzpatrick's Color Atlas and Synopsis of Clinical Dermatology, 5th ed. New York: McGraw-Hill, 2005: 5.)

a. An antibacterial cleanser
b. A topical retinoid such as tretinoin (Retin-A)
c. A topical antibiotic such as erythromycin or clindamycin (Em-gel or Cleocin)
d. An oral antibiotic such as cephalexin (Keflex)
e. A mild-potency nonfluorinated topical steroid

290. You are treating a 16-year-old girl who is complaining of severe nodular acne. She has tried and failed topical retinoids and oral antibiotics, and you are considering using isotretinoin (Accutane). Which of the following is a significant side effect that warrants discontinuing the medication?

a. Depression
b. Worsening of acne
c. Dry skin
d. Joint aches
e. Pregnancy

√**291.** You are caring for a 34-year-old woman who complains of a chronic "blush" around her cheeks and nose. Her picture is below:

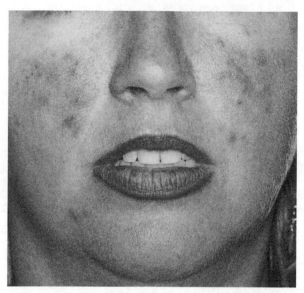

(Reproduced, with permission, from Wolff K, Johnson RA, Suurmond D. Fitzpatrick's Color Atlas and Synopsis of Clinical Dermatology, 5th ed. New York: McGraw-Hill, 2005: 9.)

Which of the following is true of this condition?

a. It has a pathogenesis similar to acne vulgaris.
b. About 50% of patients with this condition also have eye involvement.
c. Topical corticosteroids are the treatment of choice.
d. Oral therapy with tetracyclines should be reserved as a last resort.
e. Treatment should be aimed at reducing colonization of *Propionibacterium acnes*.

292. A patient comes to you with concerns about a nodule he has had on the side of his nose for several months. The nodule is shown below:

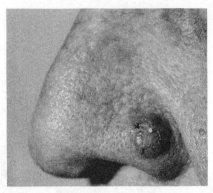

(Reproduced, with permission, from Wolff K, Johnson RA, Suurmond D. Fitzpatrick's Color Atlas and Synopsis of Clinical Dermatology, 5th ed. New York: McGraw-Hill, 2005:283.)

Which of the following is the most likely diagnosis?

a. Verruca vulgaris
b. Molluscum contagiosum
c. Nodular basal cell carcinoma
d. Squamous cell carcinoma
e. Cutaneous T-cell lymphoma

293. You are caring for a 28-year-old man who presents with a rash. A picture of his rash is shown below:

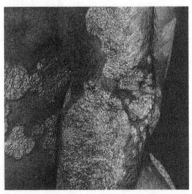

(Reproduced, with permission, from Wolff K, Johnson RA, Suurmond D. Fitzpatrick's Color Atlas and Synopsis of Clinical Dermatology, 5th ed. New York: McGraw-Hill, 2005: 59.)

He also has fingernail changes shown below:

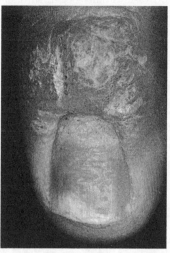

(Reproduced, with permission, from Wolff K, Johnson RA, Suurmond D. Fitzpatrick's Color Atlas and Synopsis of Clinical Dermatology, 5th ed. NewYork: McGraw-Hill, 2005:993.)

Which of the following is the most commonly prescribed therapeutic agent for his rash?

a. Oral Penicillin
b. Topical erythromycin
c. Topical pimecrolimus (Elidel)
d. Vitamin A
e. Topical corticosteroids

294. You are talking with a 24-year-old man who reports an outbreak of a mildly pruritic rash. The rash initially began with a large pink patch on his chest, to the left of his sternum breast. About a week later, he noted a more generalized eruption. The rash is shown below:

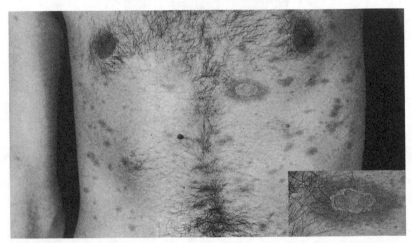

(Reproduced, with permission, from Wolff K, Johnson RA, Suurmond D. Fitzpatrick's Color Atlas and Synopsis of Clinical Dermatology, 5th ed. New York: McGraw-Hill, 2005:119.)

Which of the following treatments is indicated?

a. Antihistamines
b. Antibiotics
c. Antivirals
d. Antifungals
e. Cyclosporine

295. You are seeing a young child whose mother brings him in with a rash. It developed on his upper lip underneath his nose. He has had cold symptoms with a runny nose recently. His picture is shown below:

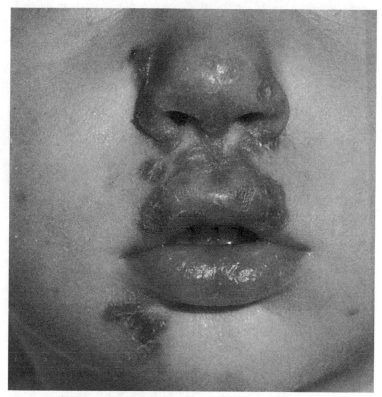

(Reproduced, with permission, from Wolff K, Johnson RA, Suurmond D. Fitzpatrick's Color Atlas and Synopsis of Clinical Dermatology, 5th ed. New York: McGraw-Hill, 2005: 589.)

Which of the following is the most likely cause of this rash?

a. Infection with group A β-hemolytic streptococci
b. Infection with *S aureus*
c. Infection with an *Enterococcus* species
d. Infection with *H influenzae*
e. Infection with a *Pseudomonas* species

296. After returning from a ski trip in the mountains, your 35-year-old patient complains of a rash for 2 days. He has multiple erythematous pustules over his legs, arms, and chest. They are not pruritic, and do not seem to be spreading. He denies any new soaps, lotions, foods, or medications. He did spend time in a hot tub on the trip. A picture of his rash is shown below:

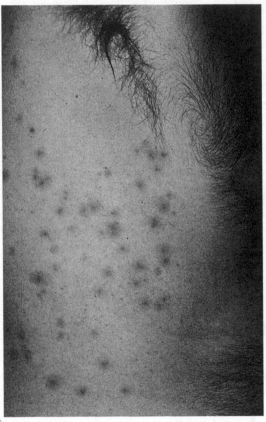

(Reproduced, with permission, from Wolff K, Johnson RA, Suurmond D. Fitzpatrick's Color Atlas and Synopsis of Clinical Dermatology, 5th ed. New York: McGraw-Hill, 2005: 982.)

Which of the following is the best treatment option for this patient?

a. Reassurance and follow up if no improvement
b. Topical steroid medication
c. Systemic steroid medication
d. Topical antibiotics with activity against *Streptococcus* and *Staphylococcus* species
e. Oral antibiotics with activity against *Pseudomonas* species

√**297.** You are seeing a 21-year-old man with a skin infection on his lip. It is the first time he has ever had this type of infection. It began with a burning at the site of the infection, then an eruption of vesicles. The rash is shown below:

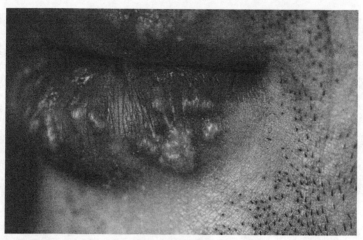

(Reproduced, with permission, from Wolff K, Johnson RA, Suurmond D. Fitzpatrick's Color Atlas and Synopsis of Clinical Dermatology, 5th ed. New York: McGraw-Hill, 2005: 803.)

Which of the following is true of this infection?

a. This is a primary infection, and future infections are likely to be more severe.
b. Based on the picture shown, distinguishing features indicate it to be a herpes simplex virus type 1 (HSV-1) infection.
c. Fever, malaise, and adenopathy are likely to be present.
d. Triggers for this rash include fever, infection, or exposure to ultraviolet light.
e. If the lesions are pustular, antibiotics are indicated.

√**298.** Your patient is known to have genital herpes. He is starting to date a new partner, and she does not have genital herpes. Which of the following statements regarding this situation is true?

a. In this case, it is recommended to use antiviral therapy only when the infection is active, but to start the medication at the first sign of an outbreak.
b. Daily therapy with an antiviral agent has been demonstrated to eliminate asymptomatic viral shedding.
c. Daily therapy with an antiviral agent can change the natural course of the infection in the affected patient.
d. Daily therapy with an antiviral agent can be associated with resistance to the antiviral medication used.
e. Daily therapy with an antiviral agent may reduce the risk of HIV transmission and acquisition.

299. An otherwise healthy 61-year-old male patient complains of a burning sensation on the posterior chest for 24 hours, and subsequent development of the rash shown below:

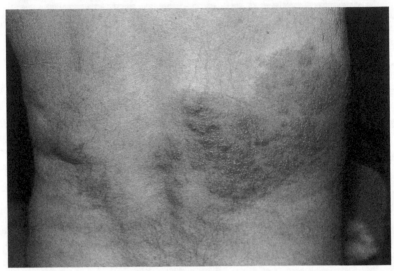

(Reproduced, with permission, from Wolff K, Johnson RA, Suurmond D. Fitzpatrick's Color Atlas and Synopsis of Clinical Dermatology, 5th ed. New York: McGraw-Hill, 2005:823.)

Which of the following is true about treatment for this condition?

a. Antiviral therapy is not indicated if the lesions have been present for more than 72 hours
b. Antiviral therapy decreases the overall duration of pain
c. Treatment with corticosteroids will decrease the likelihood of postherpetic neuralgia
d. Valacyclovir (Valtrex) is the best antiviral treatment choice for this condition
e. Antiviral resistance is common

300. You are seeing a young girl whose mother brings her in for evaluation. She has had 3 days of low-grade fever and runny nose. Today, she awakened with a rash on her cheeks, shown below:

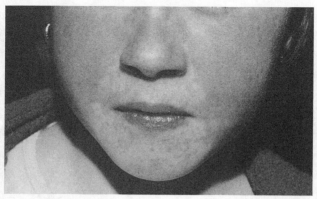

(Reproduced, with permission, from Wolff K, Johnson RA, Suurmond D. Fitzpatrick's Color Atlas and Synopsis of Clinical Dermatology, 5th ed. New York: McGraw-Hill, 2005:793.)

Which of the following is the most likely cause of her symptoms?

a. An enterovirus
b. A parvovirus
c. A parainfluenza virus
d. A varicella virus
e. Cytomegalovirus

301. You are seeing a young man who is complaining of a patch of hair loss. He denies pulling the hair, and complains that his scalp is itchy and flakey. His scalp is shown below:

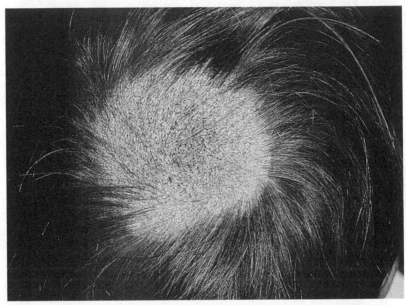

(Reproduced, with permission, from Wolff K, Johnson RA, Suurmond D. Fitzpatrick's Color Atlas and Synopsis of Clinical Dermatology, 5th ed. New York: McGraw-Hill, 2005: 709.)

Which of the following is the most effective treatment?

a. Selenium sulfide lotion, applied daily for 4 to 8 weeks
b. Ketoconazole (Nizoral) shampoo applied daily for 4 to 8 weeks
c. Clotrimazole (Lotrimin) cream, twice daily for 4 to 8 weeks
d. Griseofulvin tablets, daily for 4 to 8 weeks
e. Fluconazole (Diflucan) tablets, daily for 4 to 8 weeks

302. You are caring for a 35-year-old woman who works in a day-care. She comes to see you complaining of an itchy rash on her calf. It started as a small pink circular lesion, but is spreading. The rash is shown below:

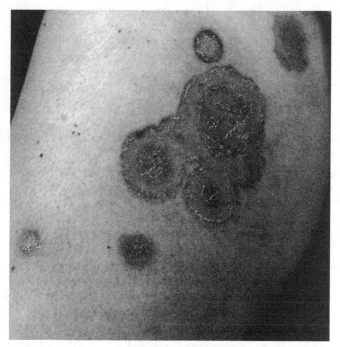

(Reproduced, with permission, from Wolff K, Johnson RA, Suurmond D. Fitzpatrick's Color Atlas and Synopsis of Clinical Dermatology, 5th ed. New York: McGraw-Hill, 2005:701.)

Which of the following is the most likely diagnosis?
a. Pityriasis rosea
b. Psoriasis
c. Tinea corporis
d. Atopic dermatitis
e. Contact dermatitis

303. A 28-year-old woman comes to you for wart removal. On examination, she has a single wart on the lateral aspect of her index finger near the distal interphalangeal joint. She has no other medical conditions, but is trying to become pregnant. Her last period was 4 weeks ago. Which of the following treatment options would be best in this situation?

a. Topical treatment with liquid nitrogen
b. Topical treatment with podophyllum resin
c. Topical treatment with local interferon inducer like Imiquimod
d. CO_2 laser treatment
e. Injection with bleomycin

304. A patient presents for evaluation of a new rash. You suspect atopic dermatitis. Which feature of the rash, if present, would lead you to suspect a different cause for the rash?

a. Lesions that are present on both antecubital areas, both cheeks, and both legs
b. Severe pruritus
c. Erythematous lesions with flaking
d. First outbreak of this rash occurring as an adult
e. Rash on the flexural surfaces of the body

305. You are caring for a 25-year-old male who presents to you for evaluation of a new lesion found on his groin. On examination you find a single small umbilicated flesh-colored papule, 4 mm in size, in his pubic region. Which of the following is true?

a. A family history of skin cancer is likely in this person
b. The patient is probably immunocompromised
c. This is likely to be a sexually transmitted infection
d. This can be spread through aerosolized droplets
e. Treatment for this condition must be surgical

306. A 32-year-old mother of two young children presents to your office for evaluation of her left eye. She reports redness of the white part of her eye, with a watery discharge. She reports mild itching and a sensation as if something is in her eye. She denies a history of allergies, and reports no concurrent allergic symptoms. Examination reveals a palpable preauricular lymph node. Fluorescein staining does not reveal corneal dendrites. Which of the following should be the treatment of choice in this case?

a. Antiviral eye drops
b. Antibacterial eye drops
c. Corticosteroid eye drops
d. Combination antibiotic/corticosteroid eye drops
e. Supportive care

307. You are seeing a 26-year-old male patient complaining of a red eye who says, "I think I have pink eye." He reports increased redness, tearing, discharge, photophobia, and pain. Which of his reported symptoms would be more suggestive of something other than conjunctivitis?

a. Redness
b. Tearing
c. Discharge
d. Photophobia
e. Pain

308. You are seeing a 20-year-old college student who reports that her eye became pink over the last 24 hours. She is otherwise healthy and takes no medications except oral contraceptives. She reports redness, irritation, tearing, discharge, and itching. Which of her symptoms are more specific for an allergic etiology for her condition?

a. Use of oral contraceptives
b. Irritation
c. Tearing
d. Discharge
e. Itching

309. You are caring for a 3-year-old boy who goes to day care while his parents are at work. His mother brought him to see you because the day care will not take him back until he's had a doctor evaluate his eye symptoms. He developed an acute redness of the left eye, associated with runny nose, cough, and increased irritability. On examination, his eye is red and watery. The discharge is clear, and he has mild eyelid edema. Which of the following is the most common cause for his condition?

a. Coxsackie virus
b. Parainfluenza virus
c. Adenovirus
d. Rhinovirus
e. Herpesvirus

310. You are seeing a 32-year-old contact lens wearer who has had several episodes of conjunctivitis in the past year. He currently complains of similar symptoms for 24 hours. Which of the following treatments would be best in this situation?

a. Supportive care
b. Ciprofloxacin (Ciloxan) ointment
c. Polymyxin-trimethoprim (Polytrim) ointment
d. Gentamicin (Garamycin) ointment
e. Immediate ophthalmologic referral

311. You are evaluating a 19-year-old college student who complains of an acute red eye. He complains that his eye feels irritated. He denies vision loss, but reports a great deal of discharge. When you wipe his eye with a tissue, the discharge reappears almost instantaneously. Which of the following statements is true?

a. This is a viral process
b. This is an allergic process
c. This is likely due to a sexually transmitted infection
d. This should be treated with oral antibiotics
e. This should be treated with topical steroids

312. You have been treating a 43-year-old woman with rheumatoid arthritis for years. You and her rheumatologist have had her illness in relatively good control. She presents to you with a red eye and significant eye pain. She denies trauma. Upon further questioning, she complains of decreased vision and headache. She describes the pain as deep and boring. Her examination reveals diffuse injection of the deeper vessels with minimal discharge. Her pupils react normally. Which of the following is her most likely diagnosis?

a. Scleritis
b. Episcleritis
c. Corneal abrasion
d. Acute glaucoma
e. Iritis

313. You are caring for a 32-year-old female smoker with upper respiratory symptoms. She reports congestion, facial pressure, nasal discharge, tooth pain, and headache. Her symptoms have been present for 14 days. Which portion of her history is most commonly used to define clinical rhinosinusitis?

a. Facial pressure
b. Nasal discharge
c. Tooth pain
d. Headache
e. Fourteen days of illness

314. A 36-year-old man has had recurrent bouts of sinusitis. He develops at least three sinus infections per year, and wants to discuss prevention. Which of the following conditions, if controlled, would be likely to decrease his recurrence rate?

a. Allergic rhinitis
b. GERD
c. Cigarette smoking
d. Environmental pollutants
e. Immunodeficiency

315. You are seeing a 21-year-old college student who complains of congestion, headache, sinus pressure, and tooth pain for more than 2 weeks. She is otherwise healthy, but feels like she's "having trouble shaking this cold." She has used over-the-counter decongestants with limited relief. A CT scan of her sinuses demonstrates acute sinusitis. Which of the following is the most common organism causing her symptoms?

a. *Moraxella catarrhalis*
b. *Staphylococcus aureus*
c. Group A β-hemolytic streptococcal species
d. *Streptococcus pneumoniae*
e. A polymicrobial mixture of many organisms

316. You are caring for a 42-year-old woman with a persistent sinusitis. She first came to see you 3 months ago, was treated with amoxicillin, and improved. She returned 2 months ago, received another course of amoxicillin, and improved again. Last month, her symptoms reoccurred, and you prescribed trimethoprim/sulfamethoxazole. She returns today with continued symptoms. Which of the following should be your treatment of choice?

a. A macrolide for 10 days
b. A macrolide for 14 to 21 days
c. A fluoroquinolone for 10 days
d. A fluoroquinolone for 14 to 21 days
e. A second- or third-generation cephalosporin for 10 days

317. You are treating a woman with chronic and recurrent sinusitis. Along with antibiotic therapy directed at the underlying bacterial cause, which of the following has been shown to help break the cycle of recurrent disease?

a. Echinacea
b. Phenylpropanolamine
c. Pseudoephedrine
d. Topical α-agonists (Afrin)
e. Topical nasal steroids

318. You are seeing a 16-year-old high school football player to discuss a recent injury. Last night, during football practice, he felt an acute numbness and tingling from his neck down to his right hand, "like an electric shock." The inciting event occurred when he was tackled, compressing his head, while his head and neck were flexed toward the right side. The numbness resolved within a few minutes, but he did not continue play. He is seeing you for evaluation and treatment. He currently has normal range of motion, with no neurological deficit or pain. Which of the following is the most appropriate next step?

a. Return to play without restriction
b. Immobilization until radiographs can be obtained
c. Immobilization until MRI can be obtained
d. Obtain an electromyelogram of the right arm before allowing return to play
e. Refer for physical therapy

319. You are working with the team physician at a local high school. One of the football players was hit with his arm extended, causing a left shoulder injury. On examination, he has acromioclavicular (AC) joint swelling, bruising, and pain. X-rays show more than a 50% AC joint separation with a posterior displacement of the clavicle. Which of the following is the best management plan for this injury?

a. Return to play when the pain subsides
b. Immobilization with a sling, and return to play when the pain subsides
c. Immobilization with a sling, and early range of motion exercises with return to play when the pain subsides
d. Reduction under conscious sedation, then immobilization, early range of motion exercises, and return to play when the pain subsides
e. Refer to orthopedic surgery

320. A 20-year-old college basketball player comes to your office complaining of knee pain. Her symptoms started several weeks ago, but she was able to play through the pain. She reports anterior knee pain, some mild swelling after activity, and significant stiffness and pain after she's been sitting for a long period of time. Examination reveals a positive patellar grind test. Based on her history and examination, which of the following exercises would be most likely to help her symptoms?

a. Patellar tendon stretching
b. Quadriceps stretching
c. Vastus lateralis strengthening
d. Vastus medialis strengthening
e. Hamstring strengthening

321. A patient comes to see you after a skiing accident 6 days ago. He reports twisting his knee during a fall, feeling a "pop," and noting significant immediate swelling. He was able to bear weight immediately, but did not ski for the rest of the trip. His pain is now improved, and he is ambulating, but he says the knee feels unstable. Which of the following is the most likely cause of his symptoms?

a. Patellofemoral pain syndrome
b. Anterior cruciate ligament (ACL) tear
c. Posterior cruciate ligament (PCL) tear
d. Meniscal injury
e. Collateral ligament tear

322. One of your patients injured his knee playing soccer. In trying to determine the extent of his injury, you palpate the joint line with one hand and internally/externally rotate while flexing and extending the knee. This maneuver elicits a catch with pain at the joint line. Which of the following knee injuries is most likely?

a. Patellar tendon rupture
b. Patellar fracture
c. ACL tear
d. Meniscal tear
e. Collateral ligament tear

323. You are seeing a 14-year-old girl who hurt her ankle while dancing yesterday. She reports that her ankle "twisted in" causing immediate pain and the inability to bear weight. In the office, she has bruising and tenderness over the anterior talofibular ligament (ATFL) with acute swelling. She is unable to bear weight due to the pain. Which of the following is the most appropriate next step?

a. Obtain x-rays of her ankle
b. Encourage early mobilization
c. Prescribe rest, ice, compression, and elevation
d. Use a NSAID to help with the pain and inflammation
e. Begin physical therapy

324. You are seeing a 56-year-old man who reports a recent syncopal episode. Which of the following tests is always indicated in the workup?

a. CBC
b. TSH assessment
c. ECG
d. Echocardiogram
e. Tilt table testing

325. A 21-year-old generally healthy college student is seeing you in your office after having "passed out" playing basketball. This has never happened before. He has no significant past medical history and takes no medications. On examination, you note a harsh crescendo-decrescendo systolic murmur, heard best at the apex and radiating to the axilla. Which of the following tests is most likely to reveal the etiology of his syncopal episode?

a. Echocardiogram
b. Holter monitoring
c. ECG
d. Stress testing
e. Tilt table testing

326. You are caring for a 49-year-old type 2 diabetic woman who presents to you after passing out. The event occurred 1 day ago, while she was walking up steps to her seat at a movie theatre. She reports that she felt breathless, became hot and sweaty, and the next thing she remembers, she was waking up on the floor. Her diabetes has been fairly well-controlled with metformin, and her last glycosolated hemoglobin 1 month ago was 7.9%. Her examination is benign, as is her ECG. Which of the following tests would be most likely to reveal the cause of her syncope?

a. Serum glucose assessment
b. Hemoglobin A1C
c. Echocardiogram
d. Stress testing
e. Twenty-four hour Holter monitoring

✓ **327.** You are evaluating a 28-year-old woman who has had several episodes of passing out. In general, the events are unpredictable, and are not preceded by any prodrome. Her examination has been consistently normal. Initial workup, including a pregnancy test, hematocrit, serum glucose, orthostatic blood pressures, and ECG were normal. She underwent 24-hour Holter monitoring and long-term ambulatory loop ECG evaluation, both of which were negative. Which of the following is the most appropriate next test?

a. Psychiatric evaluation
b. Carotid Doppler
c. MRI of the brain
d. Stress testing
e. Tilt table testing

✓ **328.** You are evaluating a 20-year-old woman complaining of vaginal discharge. She reports vaginal itch and white discharge. She has no history of vaginal infections in the past, and has never been sexually active. A potassium hydroxide (KOH) preparation of the discharge is shown below:

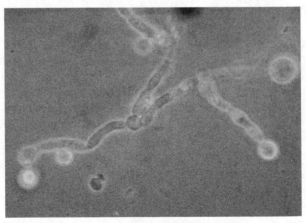

(Reproduced, with permission, from Wolff K, Johnson RA, Suurmond D. Fitzpatrick's Color Atlas and Synopsis of Clinical Dermatology, 5th ed. New York: McGraw-Hill, 2005:717.)

Which of the following is the best treatment option for this condition?

a. Reassurance that this is a normal variation and that no treatment is necessary
b. Topical azole applications
c. Topical metronidazole
d. Oral clindamycin
e. Doxycycline

√**329.** You are discussing recurrent vaginal discharge with a patient. She has been evaluated three times in the last 6 months, and has had a vaginal candidiasis each time. She has symptom-free intervals, but the infection seems to be recurrent. She is monogamous, sexually active with a male partner, takes birth control pills, and denies other complaints or known illnesses. Which of the following is most likely to improve this patient's condition?

a. Test her for diabetes, and control her elevated glucose level.
b. Ask her to discontinue her birth control pills.
c. Treat her sexual partner.
d. Test her for HIV, and begin therapy.
e. Ask her to add fiber to her diet.

√**330.** You are seeing a 17-year-old girl who reports intense vaginal itching and urinary frequency. She has been sexually active for 6 months. On examination, you note frothy yellow-green discharge with bright red vaginal mucosa and red macules on the cervix. What is the saline preparation of the discharge most likely to show?

a. Sheets of epithelial cells "studded" with bacteria
b. "Moth-eaten" epithelial cells
c. Motile triangular organisms with long tails
d. Many white blood cells
e. Hyphae

331. Your patient describes a recent vaginal discharge. She reports more discharge than usual, and an unusual odor after intercourse with her husband. A KOH preparation of the discharge produces a fishy odor, and a saline preparation is shown below:

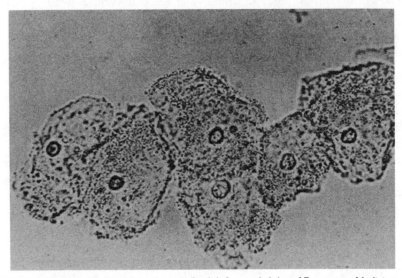

(Reproduced, with permission, from Knoop K, Stack L, Storrow A. Atlas of Emergency Medicine, 2nd ed. New York:McGraw-Hill, 2002:683.)

Which of the following is the treatment of choice for her condition?
a. Metronidazole
b. Doxycycline
c. Clotrimazole
d. Imiquimod
e. Acyclovir

332. You are caring for an 18-month-old infant, whose mother brings him in for "wheezing." She reports that he has had a runny nose and a slight cough for 2 days, along with a low-grade fever. On examination, he does not appear to be in respiratory distress, but his lung examination does reveal bilateral wheezing. Which of the following is the most likely diagnosis?
a. Acute viral respiratory tract infection
b. Pneumonia
c. Bronchiolitis
d. Aspiration
e. Asthma

333. A 61-year-old man comes to see you for shortness of breath. He has a history of hypertension, type 2 diabetes, and hyperlipidemia. He quit smoking 4 years ago after a more than 30-pack/year history. On physical examination, he is not in respiratory distress, but he has diffuse wheezing in the bilateral lower lobes of his lungs. His cardiac examination demonstrates an S_4, and he demonstrates JVD. Which of the following treatments would likely relieve his symptoms?

a. Antibiotic therapy
b. Epinephrine
c. Steroid therapy
d. Diuretics
e. Anticoagulation

334. You are seeing a 24-year-old woman who presents to your office complaining of "wheezing." She reports acute shortness of breath that occurred while she was shopping, and her wheezing is associated with pleuritic pain. She is otherwise healthy, only taking oral contraceptives. On examination, she is tachypneic, but not in acute distress. Auscultation of her lungs is normal. After the appropriate diagnostic workup, what is the best treatment option for this patient?

a. Reassurance and observation
b. Antibiotic therapy
c. Anticoagulation
d. Bronchodilators
e. Steroids

335. You are seeing a 23-year-old man for shortness of breath. He has no history of asthma or wheezing, and is otherwise healthy. His lung examination does reveal significant wheezing bilaterally. Which of the following tests is necessary?

a. Observation and treatment
b. Chest x-ray
c. Peak flow testing
d. Pulmonary function tests
e. CBC

336. You are evaluating a 9-month-old child with recurrent wheezing. His mother also reports that he vomits after formula as well. Which of the following is the best test to determine the cause of his wheezing?

a. Pulmonary function testing
b. Chest x-ray
c. Upper GI barium swallow
d. Upper endoscopy
e. Twenty-four hour pH probe

337. You are evaluating a 35-year-old patient with known asthma. He comes to your office complaining of increased shortness of breath despite compliance with his usual asthma regimen. He reports cough, but denies fever or sputum production. His pulmonary examination reveals wheezing bilaterally without crackles or rhonchi. Which of the following is most useful in this setting?

a. Chest x-ray
b. Peak flow testing
c. Pulmonary function testing
d. CBC
e. Nasopharyngeal washing

Acute Complaints

Answers

93. The answer is b. (*South-Paul, pp 310-328.*) The first priority when evaluating abdominal pain is to determine whether the pain is acute or chronic. Sudden and/or severe onset of pain should lead the clinician toward an emergent evaluation. Right lower quadrant pain is suspicious for an acute appendicitis, but by itself is not specific enough to warrant an emergent workup. A "gnawing" sensation is often described with ulcer disease, while pain that worsens after eating is associated with many conditions—pancreatitis, gallbladder disease, or even reflux. In the absence of hemodynamic instability, those causes are less likely to warrant emergent workup. Emesis with pain is not enough, by itself, to warrant emergent workup.

94. The answer is c. (*South-Paul, pp 310-328.*) The location and radiation of pain is often helpful in determining the cause of abdominal pain. Pain from an acute appendicitis usually starts in the periumbilical region before moving to the right lower quadrant. Pancreatitis generally settles in the midepigastric region with radiation to the back. Gallbladder pain is typically in the epigastric or right upper quadrant and radiates to the scapula. Esophageal spasm is often referred higher in the chest. GERD is mid-epigastric and generally does not radiate.

95. The answer is b. (*South-Paul, pp 310-328.*) Advanced age can change the presentation and perception of abdominal pain. In fact, studies estimate that there is a 10% to 20% reduction in the perceived intensity of the pain per decade after the age of 60. Only 22% of elderly patients with appendicitis present with classic symptoms, making the diagnosis more difficult. Therefore, a high index of suspicion is necessary. Small-bowel obstruction and constipation may cause bilateral lower quadrant pain and decreased appetite, but fever indicates something different. IBS is chronic and generally not associated with fever. Pancreatitis is associated with food intolerance but the associated pain is usually in the epigastric region.

96. The answer is c. (*South-Paul, pp 310-328.*) The specific site of tenderness is classic for many sources of abdominal pain. Sudden cessation of inspiratory effort during deep palpation of the right upper quadrant is called "Murphy sign" and is suggestive of acute cholecystitis. Hepatitis and gallstones may cause right upper quadrant tenderness, but generally do not elicit Murphy sign. Pain caused by pancreatitis often radiates to the back. Pain from renal calculi often radiates to the shoulder.

97. The answer is c. (*South-Paul, pp 310-328.*) The patient describes the classic presentation for peptic ulcer disease. Infection with *H pylori* is the leading cause of peptic ulcer disease, with the use of NSAIDs the second most common cause. Alcoholism and gallstones can cause pancreatitis, but that presents differently. Gastroparesis may cause dyspepsia, but is a less likely cause for ulcer disease.

98. The answer is a. (*South-Paul, pp 310-328.*) Reflux can be appropriately diagnosed by medical history and by evaluating the response to treatment. Those who respond are likely to have the diagnosis. Upper endoscopy fails to reveal GERD in 36% to 50% of the patients who have been found to have GERD by a pH probe. EGD should be performed if bleeding, weight loss, or dysphagia is present, especially in an elderly patient. The other tests have not been shown to be sensitive or specific enough to replace response to treatment as a diagnostic tool.

99. The answer is b. (*South-Paul, pp 310-328.*) In many cases of GERD, the diagnosis can be made using the medical history and trying treatment to assess for response. Symptomatic improvement after treatment is indicative of GERD, and further workup is usually unnecessary. However, endoscopy should always be performed if alarm symptoms are present. These symptoms include bleeding, abdominal mass, weight loss, dysphagia, or vomiting, especially if these symptoms are present in an elderly patient.

100. The answer is d. (*South-Paul, pp 310-328.*) ERCP is the gold standard for diagnosis and treatment of choledocholithiasis, and is usually performed in the setting of an acute cholecystitis with increased liver enzymes, amylase, or lipase. Ultrasound shows stones, but is less sensitive for choledocholithiasis or for complications (abscess, perforation, and pancreatitis). CT or MRI is better for those. Cholescintigraphy can be used, and a negative test rules out cholecystitis, but in the setting of increased liver enzymes, an ERCP is a better choice.

101. The answer is a. (*South-Paul, pp 310-328. McPhee, pp 604-607.*) The patient described in this question has pancreatitis. Gallstones cause the majority of cases of pancreatitis. Alcohol causes about 30% of the cases. Ten to thirty percent are idiopathic. Less common causes include hypercalcemia, hyperlipidemia, abdominal trauma, medications, infections, and instrumentation (for instance, after an ERCP).

102. The answer is c. (*South-Paul, pp 310-328.*) Amylase is sensitive, but not specific. Lipase is also sensitive, but more specific, as virtually all lipase is pancreatic in origin. If it is more than three times normal, it is very sensitive and specific. WBC count, glucose, and transaminases can be elevated, but are better used to assess prognosis, not make the diagnosis.

103. The answer is b. (*South-Paul, pp 310-328.*) Ranson's criteria assess the severity and prognosis of pancreatitis. On admission, 5 criteria are considered. It is a poor prognostic sign if the age is more than 55, WBC is greater than 16,000/mm^3, glucose is greater than 200 mg/dL, LDH is greater than 350 IU/L, and AST is greater than 250 U/L. Six other criteria reflect the development of complications and include a decrease in hematocrit greater than 10 mg/dL, a BUN increase greater than 5 mg/dL, calcium less than 8 mg/dL, Pao$_2$ less than 60 mm Hg, base deficit greater than 4 mEq/L and a fluid sequestration greater than 6 L. These are assessed during the first 48 hours of admission.

104. The answer is e. (*South-Paul, pp 310-328.*) IBS is typified by symptoms of abdominal pain or discomfort associated with disturbed defecation. The Rome Consensus Committee for IBS developed diagnostic criteria that are symptom, not laboratory-based. The criteria include symptoms that are present for at least 12 weeks (not necessarily consecutive) in the previous 12 months, and pain that is characterized by two of the following three features: (1) relieved by defecation, (2) onset is associated with a change in stool frequency, or (3) onset is associated with a change in the form or appearance of stool. Since the patient in this question meets criteria, laboratory testing is not necessary, but some clinicians would be reassured by a normal CBC and ESR.

105. The answer is d. (*Mahadevan, pp 145-159.*) The patient is presenting with symptoms consistent with obstruction. In this case, abdominal radiographs are crucial in the decision-making process, and to rule in/rule out a surgical abdomen. A fecalith is a hard, stony mass of feces that can obstruct the appendix or a diverticuli. Without a fever or other evidence of appendicitis, that would be a less likely finding. In a perforation, x-ray would show free intraperitoneal air, but this patient's presentation is more consistent with obstruction. Stool may be seen on an abdominal film, but constipation would not likely present with the symptoms listed above. Gallstones are less likely to be seen on plain film.

106. The answer is e. *(South-Paul, pp 310-328.)* Dyspepsia refers to a set of symptoms that can encompass a variety of diseases and the etiologies associated with them. Most clinicians describe dyspepsia as chronic or recurrent discomfort centered around the upper abdomen. Dyspepsia can be associated with heartburn, belching, bloating, nausea, or vomiting, and while common causes include peptic ulcer disease (PUD) and GERD, no specific etiology is found for 50% to 60% of patients who present with dyspepsia. Only 15% to 25% of patients with dyspepsia have ulcer disease, and only 5% to 15% have GERD. Rare causes include gastric or pancreatic cancers.

107. The answer is d. *(Mengel, pp 9-12.)* Many types of cervical and vaginal abnormalities can be detected using the Pap smear. When the results are reported as "atypical squamous cells of undetermined significance" (ASCUS), the physician may repeat the test in 4 to 6 months and in 1 year, perform HPV testing on the sample, or proceed to colposcopy. If the HPV testing is negative, the patient is at low risk for cancer, and the Pap test can be repeated in 1 year, especially if the patient is monogamous.

108. The answer is d. *(Mengel, pp 9-12.)* When the results of a Pap smear are reported as ASCUS, and HPV testing on the sample is positive, the physician should proceed to colposcopy. Colposcopy involves cervical examination under stereoscopic magnification and includes biopsy of abnormal-appearing areas, and is the definitive test for assessing Pap smear abnormalities. Imiquimod (Aldara) is an immune modulator and can treat warts, but is not indicated in this case.

109. The answer is c. *(Mengel, pp 9-12.)* When the results of a Pap smear are reported as ASCUS, and HPV testing is unavailable, the physician may choose to perform colpscopy or repeat the Pap smear in 4 to 6 months. If the physician chooses to repeat the Pap smear, the results should be carefully followed. If the results are reported as ASCUS or higher, a colposcopy should be performed. If the repeat is normal, the Pap should be repeated again in 4 to 6 months. If the repeat Pap smear is again negative, the frequency of testing can return to normal.

110. The answer is d. (*Mengel, pp 9-12.*) When the results of a Pap smear are reported as ASCUS, favoring low-grade squamous intraepithelial lesion (LSIL), the physician should proceed to colposcopy. Colposcopy involves cervical examination under stereoscopic magnification and includes biopsy of abnormal appearing areas, and is the definitive test for assessing Pap smear abnormalities. If the biopsies confirm the diagnosis, definitive treatment is needed.

111. The answer is d. (*Mengel, pp 9-12.*) When the results of a Pap smear are reported as "atypical glandular cells," the physician should proceed to colposcopy. Colposcopy involves endocervical sampling, and will help to further identify the glandular cell abnormality noted on the Pap smear.

112. The answer is e. (*Mengel, pp 9-12.*) When the results of a Pap smear are reported as atypical glandular cells, and are reported to be of endometrial origin, endometrial biopsy is necessary to rule out endometrial cancer. This is true even if the patient does not report abnormal vaginal bleeding.

113. The answer is a. (*South-Paul, pp 329-342.*) Iron deficiency may be asymptomatic, but patients may present with varying degrees of weakness, fatigue, dizziness, palpitations, or exercise intolerance. On physical examination, one may see pallor and tachycardia. Pica, the craving of ice, clay, or other substances is particularly associated with iron deficiency. Lead, anemia of chronic disease, vitamin B_{12}, and folate deficiency usually do not cause pica.

114. The answer is c. (*McPhee, pp 422-438.*) Anemias can often be classified by cell size. Causes of microcytic anemias include iron deficiency, anemia of chronic disease, thalassemia, and sideroblastic anemias. In iron deficiency, the red cell distribution width (RDW) would be elevated due to variation in cell size. In sideroblastic anemia, the MCV would be normal, high, or low, but the red cells are dimorphic. In thalassemia, the RDW would be normal because the red cells are uniformly small. Aplastic anemia and anemia due to chronic renal insufficiency are generally normocytic.

115. The answer is a. (*South-Paul, pp 329-342.*) The laboratory evaluation in this patient clearly indicates iron deficiency anemia. The most common cause is blood loss. Poor nutrition and/or inadequate absorption are less common causes. Chronic disease would lead to a high or normal ferritin and a low TIBC. Folic acid deficiency would lead to an elevated MCV.

116. The answer is e. (*South-Paul, pp 329-342.*) The laboratory results indicate anemia of chronic illness, in this case lupus. It is likely a result of trapping of iron stores in the reticuloendothelial system, mild decrease in erythropoietin production and decreased marrow response to erythropoietin. Although iron therapy and erythropoietin may help slightly, the mainstay of his treatment is treating the underlying condition. Transfusions may be necessary preoperatively if the hemoglobin is less than 10 mg/dL.

117. The answer is d. (*South-Paul, pp 329-342.*) The patient described has a laboratory profile suspicious for thalassemia minor. These patients have low hemoglobin and MCV, but in contrast to iron deficiency, the patients have an elevated RBC and normal RDW. Additionally, the MCV is low out of proportion to the anemia. Given that the patient is asymptomatic, he should be treated only if necessary. Treatment includes transfusion if blood loss leads to significant anemia. The patient should have genetic counseling if planning a family.

118. The answer is c. (*South-Paul, pp 329-342.*) Some clinical features are common to all megaloblastic anemias—anemia, pallor, weight loss, fatigue, and glossitis to name a few. Neurological symptoms are specific to vitamin B_{12} deficiency. Usually, treatment is parenteral vitamin B_{12} replacement weekly for 1 month, often with concurrent administration of folic acid. Once levels are established, oral therapy may be sufficient.

119. The answer is e. (*South-Paul, pp 329-342.*) Most often, vitamin B_{12} deficiency is a result of inadequate absorption. Since vitamin B_{12} is present in all animal products, only strict vegans or people not ingesting animal products would be deficient from a dietary standpoint. Vitamin B_{12} deficiency is not a side effect of hydrochlorothiazide. Alcohol can impact intracellular processing of folic acid, but not vitamin B_{12}.

120. The answer is b. (*South-Paul, pp 329-342.*) The slide shows sicklecell anemia, an autosomal recessive trait seen in those of African, Mediterranean, or Asian heritage. It is found before the age of 6 in 90% of patients, with acute pain crises as the most common presentation. Prophylaxis for pain crises involves ensuring adequate oxygenation and hydration. Immunization against streptococcal infection is appropriate, as most patients are functionally asplenic. The patients often have daily prophylaxis with penicillin until the age of 5. Immunization and antibiotic prophylaxis does not, however, prevent pain crises. Chronic analgesics and scheduled transfusions have not been shown to reduce pain crises.

121. The answer is b. *(Mengel, pp 37-43.)* The skin lesions of Rocky Mountain spotted fever are typically red macules on peripheral extremities that become purpuric and confluent. Lyme disease typically presents as a slowly spreading anular lesion—erythema chronicum migrans. Tularemia is characterized by pain and ulceration at the bite site. Brown recluse spider bites most often present as local pain and itching, then a hemorrhagic bulla with surrounding erythema and induration. The black widow bite is characterized by a mild prick followed by pain at the bite site.

122. The answer is a. *(Mengel, pp 37-43.)* Lyme disease occurs in the New England states, New York, and Wisconsin, but can be seen sporadically in the west and in other midwest areas. Rocky Mountain spotted fever occurs in the western mountain states, Tularemia in the west, brown recluse spider bites in the south central United States, and chiggers in the southern and midwestern United States.

123. The answer is c. *(Mengel, pp 37-43.)* This case describes the typical presentation and physical examination findings of head lice, including the typical erythematous popular rash and "nits" on the hair follicles. Fleas, bedbugs, scabies, and chiggers may all present with erythematous papules, but would have a different distribution and would not have associated nits.

124. The answer is d. *(Mengel, pp 37-43.)* This case describes the classic distribution of scabies. Sarcoptes scabiei burrow into intertriginous areas, wrists, or areas where clothing is tight next to the skin. The lesions of chigger bites are similar, but bites are typically found in a linear pattern over wrists, ankles, and legs. Bedbugs typically infest unclothed areas—the neck, hands, and face. Fleas typically bite the lower extremities, and lesions from body lice would not follow the pattern described.

125. The answer is c. *(Mengel, pp 37-43.)* After a cat bite, hospitalization is indicated only if the bite involves the tendon, joint capsule, bone, or hand.

Bites from a domestic cat carry a small risk of rabies, and immune globulin is not indicated. If rabies is suspected, the cat can be observed or tested. Treatment for the person can begin up to 8 days after exposure. Cat bites can become infected with *P multocida,* which is sensitive to amoxicillin/clavulanate, but not clindamycin. Subcutaneous sutures are not recommended when closing a bite wound, as they are more likely to become infected.

126. The answer is b. *(Rakel, pp 943-946.)* Typical local reactions to stings include swelling, erythema, and pain at and around the site of the sting. In general, they resolve quickly and minimal analgesia is all that is necessary. Large local reactions include extended areas of swelling that last several days. They are not allergic in origin, and carry a minimal risk of anaphylaxis upon reexposure. Toxic systemic reactions are associated with nausea, vomiting, headache, vertigo, syncope, convulsions, and fever. Pruritis, erythema, and urticaria are less common. Persons who have a toxic reaction are at risk for anaphylaxis with subsequent stings. The reaction described in the above question is not anaphylactic in nature.

127. The answer is a. *(Mengel, pp 44-48.)* Gynecomastia is a benign enlargement of the male breast. It may be asymptomatic or painful, bilateral or unilateral. It commonly occurs around the time of puberty, and if so, requires only a history, physical examination, and reassurance if there are no abnormalities found. Most cases resolve within 1 year. Outside of the pubertal period, assessment of hepatic, renal, and thyroid functions may help uncover a cause. Sex hormones are only tested if progressive enlargement is noted.

128. The answer is c. *(Mengel, pp 44-48.)* Fibrocystic changes are the most common benign condition of the breast. Cysts may range in size from 1 mm to more than 1 cm in size. Fibroadenomas are usually rubbery, smooth, well-circumscribed, nontender, and freely mobile. Mammograms are not necessary for women under 30 years of age, as they are less sensitive in younger women with denser breast tissue. Mastitis generally occurs with nursing, and is characterized by inflammation, edema, and erythema in areas of the breast.

129. The answer is d. *(Mengel, pp 44-48.)* Up to 15% of breast cancers are mammographically silent. Therefore, a palpable mass deserves further workup, even if the mammogram is negative. Workup may include an ultrasound to determine if the mass is cystic or solid, and possible biopsy. Aspiration of the mass may be appropriate, but biopsy is still necessary if the mass is palpable after aspiration, if the fluid is bloody, or if the mass reappears within 1 month. The characteristics of the fluid otherwise does not dictate workup. Genetic testing is of no value in the workup of a breast mass, but can be considered based on family history, and under the direction of an experienced genetic counselor.

130. The answer is e. (*Mengel, pp 44-48.*) Patients with mastitis should be encouraged to continue nursing, and should be started on an antibiotic that covers *streptococcal* and staphylococcal infections. Reducing caffeine and methylxanthines, or using evening primrose oil may decrease symptoms of fibrocystic breast disease, but has no impact on mastitis. Applying heat may help symptoms, but ice will not have the desired effect.

131. The answer is a. (*Mengel, pp 44-48.*) Spontaneous, unilateral discharge is most suspicious for breast cancer. The characteristics of the discharge cannot be used to distinguish benign versus malignant causes, however, bloody, serous, serosanguineous, or watery discharge deserve a workup.

132. The answer is c. (*Mengel, pp 44-48.*) The degree of abnormality seen on a mammogram is classified using the breast imaging reporting and data system (BI-RADS). BI-RADS classification 0 means that the test was incomplete, and additional testing should be conducted as soon as possible. BI-RADS 1 and 2 mean that the mammogram is benign, and routine screening can be conducted at usual intervals. BI-RADS 3 indicates that the lesion is probably benign, but that diagnostic mammogram should be performed in 6 months. BI-RADS 4 and 5 are suspicious for, and highly suggestive of, cancer (respectively) and that tissue diagnosis is needed.

133. The answer is c. (*McPhee, pp 613-632.*) MRI imaging is being evaluated as a method to screen for breast cancer. It is highly sensitive, but not specific, and should not be used as a general screening test for breast cancer. However, it can be useful in selected high-risk women (eg, those with breast cancer genetic mutations). At this time, it is not generally accepted for use to clarify suspicious mammographic or ultrasonographic findings except when examining the contralateral breast in a woman with known cancer, or to evaluate the extent of a lobular carcinoma.

134. The answer is d. (*Mengel, pp 48-54.*) Hand cellulitis often follows puncture wounds, and cat bites may often produce infection with *P multocida.*

Most skin infections are due to *S aureus* or *S pyogenes*. *Clostridium perfringens* may produce gas, and should be considered as a cause for cellulitis that can lead to gangrene, especially if crepitus is found on clinical examination. *Haemophilus influenzae* sometimes infects the skin of younger children.

135. The answer is c. *(Mengel, pp 48-54.)* Hot-tub folliculitis is commonly seen in the setting described in this question. Often, the infection is self-limited, but occasionally antibiotics with pseudomonal coverage are necessary. While streptococcal and staphylococcal species are common causes of folliculitis, in the case of recent hot tub use, *Pseudomonas* is more likely. Tinea and candida do not generally cause folliculitis.

136. The answer is a. *(Rakel, pp 1021-1024.)* Tinea infections are common, and may be spread by close person-to-person contact (as in school wrestling). The classic tinea lesion is pruritic, erythematous, with raised borders, and central scaling. This can often be confused with eczema or a bacterial skin infection, but by scraping the lesion and visualizing hyphae with microscopic examination, the diagnosis of tinea can be confirmed. Tinea cruris occurs in the groin, not on the thigh, pityriasis rosea has a different classic appearance.

137. The answer is a. *(Meisel, 2006.)* When someone presents to the office complaining of chest pain, the history is invaluable in helping determine if the pain is due to a life-threatening cause (myocardial infarction, pulmonary embolism, aortic dissection, or tension pneumothorax, to name a few). Studies have shown that the likelihood of myocardial infarction with a chest pain history increases when pain is said to

- Radiate to the right, left, or both arms/shoulders
- Be exertional
- Be associated with diaphoresis
- Be associated with nausea or vomiting
- Be described as a "pressure"
- Be described as worse than previous cases of angina, or similar to past MI

The likelihood decreases when the pain is described as pleuritic.

138. The answer is c. *(Meisel, 2006.)* Historical features are important when determining likely causes of chest pain. In the case described, several of the symptoms are nonspecific, and may be related to any of several etiologies.

Shortness of breath is possible in asthma, PE, ischemia, or bronchitis. Cough is also possible in asthma, PE, and bronchitis. Pain that is worse with lying down is more commonly associated with a PE, but the key feature here is the abrupt onset. In general, musculoskeletal pain not associated with trauma has a vague onset. Pain from asthma and bronchitis is usually not abrupt. Pain from myocardial ischemia is usually gradual as well, and associated with activity.

139. The answer is c. *(Meisel, 2006.)* Nitroglycerine may relieve the pain of myocardial ischemia, but is not reliable enough to distinguish between ischemia and other noncardiac causes of chest pain. Relief of pain with a GI cocktail is similarly unreliable. If pain is relieved with eating, it is likely GI in origin, and if it is relieved with sitting up and leaning forward, pericarditis is likely. Relief with activity cessation is strongly suggestive of ischemic pain.

140. The answer is a. *(Light, 2006.)* Given his history and physical examination findings, the patient is likely to have a spontaneous pneumothorax. Of the options listed, chest tube insertion may be the most appropriate therapeutic intervention. Antibiotics, bronchodilators, anticoagulation, and aspirin may be appropriate with other diagnoses, but not in this case.

141. The answer is e. *(Meisel, 2006.)* In general, young people presenting with chest pain do not increase suspicion for myocardial ischemia, but when historical features are appropriate, it must be considered. While a family history of heart disease is a risk factor for myocardial ischemia, it is less likely in this very young patient. "Heartburn" is not a feature suggestive of myocardial ischemia. A recent viral infection may precede an episode of pericarditis or myocarditis, either of which could present with severe chest pain, but this does not increase suspicion for ischemia. His smoking history is certainly significant, but not as important as his history of drug use given his age. His physical examination findings (diaphoresis and agitation) are more consistent with a stimulant use, likely cocaine. The risk of myocardial infarction increases 24 times that of baseline in the 60 minutes after cocaine use.

142. The answer is d. *(Mengel, pp 54-60.)*Pain that is increased with palpation is most often associated with a musculoskeletal etiology. In this case, treatment with NSAIDs is most appropriate. A chest x-ray and blood work is not necessary at this time. An ECG might be indicated if there were risk factors for coronary artery disease, but based on this patient's symptoms and lack of concerning historical features, it would not be necessary. A proton pump inhibitor would not be indicated for pain that is worsened with palpation.

143. The answer is e. *(Mengel, pp 54-60.)* The ECG shown has no acute changes, but is suggestive of left ventricular hypertrophy. Her symptoms are quite suggestive of angina. Since she is currently asymptomatic and her ECG shows nothing acute, transfer to the hospital is unwarranted. The best approach would include patient education for warning signs, and some sort of stress testing. For women in her age group, stress ECGs are often falsely positive, so a stress test with imaging is most appropriate.

144. The answer is d. *(Meisel, 2006.)* The physical examination findings described, including the murmur and carotid pulse findings (pulsus parvus et tardus), are very suggestive of aortic stenosis. Syncope associated with chest pain may be seen in aortic dissection, a PE, LVH, or mitral valve prolapse, but none of these would be likely to have the classic physical examination findings described.

145. The answer is a. *(Meisel, 2006.)* Exercise ECG testing is simple and inexpensive. It is not useful in the face of an abnormal resting ECG (ST-segment changes, left ventricular hypertrophy, Wolff-Parkinson-White syndrome, or paced rhythm). Chemical stress tests or tests with imaging are reserved for those who cannot exercise or those who have baseline ECG abnormalities. Catheterization would not be indicated, and electron beam CT scanning is not clinically useful in this setting.

146. The answer is d. *(Meisel, 2006.)* According to the 2002 ACA/AHA guidelines, β-blockers should be discontinued for four to five half-lives (typically around 48 hours) prior to stress testing if possible. The drug should be withdrawn gradually. Hydrochlorothiazide does not interfere with stress testing.

147. The answer is d. *(Mengel, pp 72-81.)* The differential diagnosis for an acute cough includes asthma exacerbation, acute bronchitis, aspiration, exposure to irritants (cigarette smoke, pollutants), allergic rhinitis, uncomplicated pneumonia, sinusitis with postnasal drip, and viral upper respiratory infection. Of these usual causes, viral upper respiratory infection is by far the most common cause. Viral upper respiratory infection is the most frequent illness in humans with a prevalence of up to 35%.

148. The answer is a. *(Mengel, pp 72-81.)* The most common causes of a chronic cough are asthma, postnasal drainage, smoking, and GERD. Given that he did not respond to a bronchodilator, asthma is an unlikely diagnosis. Pertussis would have likely responded to azithromycin, and is therefore not likely to be the correct answer in this case. His sore throat, combined with symptoms that are worse when lying down, caffeine, or alcohol make GERD the most likely diagnosis. Medication side effects should be considered, with the ACE inhibitors most likely to cause a cough. The patient described is not on this class of medication.

149. The answer is b. *(Mengel, pp 72-81.)* Because the patient reports a productive cough for at least 3 months of the year for at least 2 consecutive years, she meets the criteria for chronic bronchitis. This is the most common cause of chronic cough in smokers. While it is true that her smoking may cause irritation of her airways, it wouldn't explain why the cough isn't present year-round (since she continues to smoke throughout the year). The most common cause of chronic cough in nonsmokers is postnasal drainage, but since this patient has a significant smoking history, chronic bronchitis is more likely. Lung cancers rarely present solely with cough. Associated signs and symptoms include weight loss and hemoptysis. Asthma is less likely to present with a productive cough.

150. The answer is e. *(Mengel, pp 72-81.)* The Centers for Disease Control published guidelines for treating acute bronchitis. The guidelines state that antibiotics are not indicated for uncomplicated acute bronchitis, regardless of the duration of the cough. Antibiotics should be reserved for patients with significant chronic obstructive pulmonary disease (COPD), CHF, those who are very ill-appearing or the elderly. This patient likely has hyperresponsive airways, sometimes called a postbronchitic cough. In this case, the best treatment would be an inhaled steroid or oral steroid taper. Anti-inflammatory medications and nasal steroids are not effective.

151. The answer is d. *(Mengel, pp 72-81.)* Antibiotics do not alter the course of pertussis unless initiated early in the illness. However, antibiotics do prevent transmission and decrease the need for respiratory isolation from 4 weeks to 1 week, and are therefore recommended. The first-line antibiotic choice is either erythromycin for 14 days, or azithromycin for 5 days. Amoxicillin and amoxicillin/clavulanate are not effective.

152. The answer is a. (*Mengel, pp 95-104.*) Acute diarrhea is defined as an increased number or decreased consistency of stool lasting 14 days or less. Most acute diarrhea is due to infection and usually occurs after the ingestion of contaminated food or water, or direct person-to-person contact. Viral infections account for 70% to 80% of acute infectious diarrhea, with rotavirus being the most frequent cause. Enteric adenoviruses are the second most common type. Rotavirus occurs in the winter months, and most cases occur between the ages of 3 months and 2 years. Contaminated water, salads, or shellfish may transmit Norwalk virus. Giardiasis is less common in the general population, but may be more prevalent in children in daycare centers. *Salmonella* is generally due to raw or undercooked meat, and enterotoxigenic *E coli* is the most common cause of traveler's diarrhea.

153. The answer is e. (*Mengel, pp 95-104.*) Approximately one-third of travelers to underdeveloped countries will develop travelers' diarrhea. Of those, 40% will alter their plans because of the symptoms, 20% will be bed-bound for at least 1 day, and 1% will require hospitalization. Most cases of travelers' diarrhea are due to enterotoxigenic *E coli*. The other causes of diarrhea are less likely causes in a person with a recent international travel history.

154. The answer is b. (*Mengel, pp 95-104.*) The antibiotic of choice for travelers' diarrhea is a fluoroquinolone (ciprofloxacin, ofloxacin, or norfloxacin) with trimethoprim/sulfamethoxazole or azithromycin being acceptable alternatives. The other antibiotics listed may be useful for other causes of diarrhea, but are not indicated for travelers' diarrhea.

155. The answer is e. (*Mengel, pp 95-104.*) For acute viral diarrhea, adults should be encouraged to eat potatoes, rice, wheat, noodles, crackers, bananas, yogurt, boiled vegetables, and soup. Dairy products, alcohol, and caffeine should be avoided. Oral rehydrating solutions can be used if vomiting is a problem, and fasting is not indicated. Some fruit juices can exacerbate diarrhea.

156. The answer is d. (*Mengel, pp 105-108.*) "Dizziness" is a subjective symptom, often meaning different things to different people. It is imperative that this complaint be better characterized to develop an appropriate differential diagnosis and treatment plan. Vertigo is a rotational sensation, in which the room spins around the patient. Orthostasis refers to lightheadedness upon arising, common with orthostatic hypotension. Presyncope is a feeling of impending faint. Disequilibrium is a sensation of unsteadiness, or a loss of balance. If asked whether the problem is in the head or the feet, patients often respond by saying the problem is in the feet. Lightheadedness is often vaguely described as a "floating" sensation.

157. The answer is c. (*Mengel, pp 105-108.*) Acoustic neuroma typically presents with unilateral tinnitus and hearing loss. The symptoms are constant and slowly progressive. With continued tumor growth, symptoms of vertigo, facial weakness, and ataxia can occur. Vestibular neuronitis presents with an acute onset of severe vertigo lasting several days, with symptoms improving over several weeks. Benign positional vertigo typically involves symptoms with position changes only. Meniere disease presents with discrete attacks of vertigo lasting for several hours, associated with nausea and vomiting, hearing loss, and tinnitus. A cerebellar tumor would typically present with dysequilibrium as opposed to tinnitus.

158. The answer is a. (*Mengel, pp 105-108.*) The Dix-Hallpike maneuver, described in the question, is often useful to distinguish central from peripheral causes of vertigo. With a peripheral cause of vertigo, the latency time for the onset of symptoms of vertigo or nystagmus is 3 to 10 seconds, the symptoms are severe, and the direction of the nystagmus is fixed. In addition, repeating the maneuver lessens the symptoms. With a central cause of vertigo, there is no latency to onset of symptoms, no lessening of symptoms with repeat maneuvers, the direction of the nystagmus changes, and the symptoms are of mild intensity. Of the above answers, all are peripheral causes of vertigo, except the correct answer, stroke.

159. The answer is b. (*Mengel, pp 105-108.*) Once diagnosed with a peripheral vestibular disorder, antihistamines are the first-line therapy for symptomatic relief. They suppress the vestibular end organ receptors and inhibit activation of the vagal response. Meclizine (Antivert), 25 mg orally every 4 to 6 hours and diphenhydramine (Benadryl), 50 mg orally every 4 to 6 hours are commonly recommended choices. Antiemetics may be used if nausea and vomiting are prominent symptoms. Benzodiazepines may be helpful in symptom reduction, but are usually second-line agents. NSAIDs and antibiotics are not helpful.

160. The answer is e. (*Mengel, pp 116-121.*) Those at risk for obstructive lung disease include pediatric patients (asthma, bronchitis, bronchiolitis), adults with asthma, and adults with chronic cigarette smoking. Dyspnea due to restrictive lung disease is more likely with occupational exposures (for farmers, cotton dust, grain dust, and hay mold), those with severe scoliosis, the morbidly obese, and the pregnant patients.

161. The answer is d. (*Mengel, pp 116-121.*) Guillain-Barre syndrome causes dyspnea due to respiratory muscle paralysis or dysfunction. A main clinical feature is bilateral symmetric progressive weakness after resolution of the infectious process. Parkinson disease and ALS generally present in an older population. Lyme disease can cause a polyneuropathy, but is unlikely without other symptoms. Psychogenic weakness and dyspnea is less likely with these clinical findings.

162. The answer is c. (*Mengel, pp 116-121.*) Symptoms of pneumonia include dyspnea, cough, sputum production, and occasionally pleuritic chest pain. Signs include fever, tachypnea, rales, dullness to percussion, and egophony. Asthma, PE, and CHF would be less likely to be associated with a fever, and bronchitis would be unlikely to be associated with egophony. While some pneumonias are viral in origin, egophony in the lower lobe indicates consolidation and antibiotics are the best therapeutic option.

163. The answer is e. (*Mengel, pp 116-121.*) The patient is presenting with signs and symptoms of CHF. These include abnormal heart sounds (a murmur or an additional heart sound), cardiomegaly, JVD, basilar rales, and dependent edema. Bronchodilators would be appropriate for asthma or bronchitis. Antibiotics may be appropriate for pneumonia. Steroids would be helpful with an asthma or COPD exacerbation. Anticoagulation may be appropriate for a DVT.

164. The answer is b. (*Mengel, pp 116-121.*) Asthma in children is characterized by recurrent episodes of wheezing. Bronchiolitis and pneumonia may also cause wheezing, but would be less likely to be recurrent. Congenital heart disease can also cause dyspnea and even cyanosis with exertion, but are less likely to cause wheezing.

165. The answer is a. (*Mengel, pp 116-121.*) B-type natriuretic peptide evaluates for the presence of CHF. Studies indicate that a value less than 80 pg/mL has a high (99%) negative predicative value and helps rule out CHF.

166. The answer is e. *(Mengel, pp 116-121.)* A D-dimer test is useful in determining the risk for a DVT or PE. A low result has a high negative predictive value for the presence of thrombus. If the result were high, a confirmatory test would be appropriate. A spiral CT scan has become a standard validated test. A V/Q scan, often used in the past, can be used when a spiral CT is unavailable, but is often indeterminate. A pulmonary angiogram is the gold standard. Doppler flow studies are used to verify a DVT. If positive, a PE can be assumed in the correct clinical setting.

167. The answer is d. *(Mengel, pp 116-121.)* Many studies have shown that opioids relieve dyspnea in patients with cancer, but the mechanism is unknown. Bronchodilators are better in the setting of COPD and asthma, as are steroids. Anxiolytics help, but seem to relieve the anxiety associated with dyspnea more than the dyspnea itself. Pulmonary rehabilitation would be an inappropriate step in a dying patient.

168. The answer is a. *(Mengel, pp 121-126.)* A recent meta-analysis found that four factors correlate significantly with a diagnosis of acute bacterial cystitis. They are frequency, hematuria, dysuria, and back pain. In addition, four factors decrease the likelihood of UTI (absent dysuria, absent back pain, history of vaginal discharge, and history of vaginal irritation). Women with any combination of the positive and negative symptoms have a more than 90% probability of a UTI. Urethritis is more likely with a gradual onset. Patients with pyelonephritis often have fever. Interstitial cystitis tends to be more chronic in nature, and is generally not associated with back pain. Vulvovaginitis is a common cause of dysuria, but is associated with vaginal irritation or discharge.

169. The answer is d. *(Mengel, pp 121-126.)* Four factors decrease the likelihood of a UTI. These include absent dysuria, absent back pain, history of vaginal discharge, and history of vaginal irritation. The other things listed do not decrease the likelihood of a UTI.

170. The answer is a. *(Mengel, pp 121-126.)* Urine culture is indicated when acute bacterial cystitis is suspected, but the urinalysis leaves the diagnosis in question. Therefore, in the setting of classic symptoms but a negative dipstick or microscopic evaluation, a culture will confirm the diagnosis. In the other cases, either the urine dipstick or microscopic evaluation confirms the clinical suspicion and culture is not indicated.

171. The answer is d. (*Mengel, pp 121-126.*) In 85% of women with recurrent UTIs, symptoms develop within 24 hours of sexual intercourse. If measures like voiding after intercourse, acidification of the urine, and discontinuing diaphragm do not work, prophylaxis is indicated for women with frequent infections. Single-dose postcoital antibiotic use is often helpful. If that does not decrease infections, daily single dose antibiotic prophylaxis may be appropriate for 3 to 6 months. If symptoms reoccur after discontinuation of daily prophylaxis, it may need to continue for 1 to 2 years.

172. The answer is b. (*Mengel, pp 121-126.*) Dysuria without pyuria is common. In the postmenopausal years, atrophy is a usual cause. In younger women, a careful history can reveal a bladder irritant (caffeine and acidic foods are common irritants). When hematuria is present, interstitial cystitis should be suspected. Interstitial cystitis is generally diagnosed through cystoscopy, based on the presence of ulcerations and fissures in the bladder mucosa and the absence of bladder tumors. Urodynamic studies often demonstrate a small bladder capacity, with urge to void with as little as 150 mL of fluid in the bladder.

173. The answer is b. (*Mengel, pp 121-126.*) The American College of Obstetrics and Gynecology recommends treating asymptomatic bacteriuria in pregnancy, as 20% to 35% of the cases eventually develop into overt UTIs. In the other cases above, treatment of asymptomatic bacteriuria is not indicated, as it has not been shown to decrease morbidity and may increase the likelihood of developing resistant microorganisms.

174. The answer is e. (*Mengel, pp 376-383.*) In men with urinary symptoms and a normal urinary tract, cystitis, and pyelonephritis are uncommon. Urethritis would be unlikely to cause this systemic illness. The patient described above has acute bacterial prostatitis. Acute prostatitis is most commonly seen in 30- to 50-year-old men, and symptoms include frequency, urgency, and back pain. The patient generally appears acutely ill, and has pyuria. The prostate examination would reveal a boggy, tender, and warm prostate.

175. The answer is b. (*South-Paul, pp 36-52.*) The chief risk factor for the development of otitis media in a child is day care. Other risk factors include an increased number of siblings living in the same house, exposure to tobacco smoke, pacifier use, formula feeding, and a lower socioeconomic status.

Children with abnormalities of the palatal architecture such as those with Down syndrome or cleft abnormalities are also at increased risk. Immunization against *H influenzae* and *S pneumoniae* have not had much impact on otitis media, as most infection is caused by nontypeable *Haemophilus* and by strains not covered by the pediatric 7-valent vaccine. The other things listed are not direct risk factors for the development of otitis media.

176. The answer is b. *(Mengel, pp 126-132.)* The patient has temporomandibular joint dysfunction, a common cause of referred otalgia. The first-line of therapy includes treatment with NSAIDs, heat, a mechanical soft diet, and referral to the dentist if there is no improvement in 3 to 4 weeks. Antibiotic therapy is not indicated. Obtaining an MRI would not add value to the diagnosis or treatment plan at this stage. An ESR may be elevated in temporal arteritis, another cause of referred ear pain, but would not be likely to be useful in this setting.

177. The answer is d. *(Mengel, pp 126-132. South-Paul, pp 41-65.)* A reddened tympanic membrane, by itself, is not a sufficient finding to diagnose acute otitis media. It may be due to increased intravascular pressure associated with crying. More reliable findings include an opaque tympanic membrane (indicating a purulent effusion), a bulging tympanic membrane, and impaired tympanic membrane mobility. When all three of those characteristics are present, the positive predictive value is near 90%. Purulent discharge in the ear canal may indicate a tympanic membrane perforation, and in the face of an otherwise normal canal is more indicative of acute otitis media than otitis externa.

178. The answer is a. *(Mengel, pp 126-132.)* Effusions may take up to 3 months to resolve. Antibiotics are not indicated for persistent effusions in the absence of acute otitis media. Effusions persisting beyond 3 months require evaluation by an otolaryngologist. Decongestants or antihistamines have never been documented to help effusions, but may be symptomatically helpful.

179. The answer is b. *(Mengel, pp 126-132.)* The picture represents acute otitis media. The child should be treated with a first-line antibiotic, and of those listed, amoxicillin is the best choice. Azithromycin is often used as a first-line choice in 1-day, 3-day, or 5-day doses, but it should be reserved as a second-line therapy.

180. The answer is c. *(McPhee, pp 168-180.)* Fundamental to the treatment of external otitis media is protection from additional moisture and avoidance of further mechanical injury from scratching. Otic drops containing antibiotics and corticosteroids are very effective. Oral antibiotics or steroids are rarely indicated, as the process is generally localized, not systemic, and demonstrates a good response to topical therapy.

181. The answer is c. *(Mengel, pp 132-136.)* There are many medications known to cause peripheral edema as a side effect. Antihypertensives, such as calcium channel blockers are well-known to cause this, but direct vasodilators, β-blockers, centrally acting agents, and antisympathetics also can cause edema. Of the diabetic medications, insulin sensitizers, such as rosiglitazone often cause edema. Hormones, corticosteroids, and NSAIDs also cause problems. SSRIs like fluoxetine do not commonly cause this symptom. Neither do ACE inhibitors, like lisinopril, or thiazide diuretics.

182. The answer is e. *(Mengel, pp 132-136.)* In the workup of edema, the first thing to note is if the edema is bilateral or unilateral. Bilateral edema associated with signs and symptoms of CHF (dyspnea, rales, or JVD) would necessitate a chest x-ray to rule in the diagnosis, followed by an echocardiogram. If ascites is present, liver function studies are needed. If these are absent, the clinician should check an urinalysis. If the sediment is abnormal, nephritic syndrome or acute tubular necrosis (ATN) is the likely diagnosis.

183. The answer is c. *(Mengel, pp 132-136.)* In the workup of edema, the first thing to note is if the edema is bilateral or unilateral. Bilateral edema associated with dyspnea, rales, or JVD would necessitate an evaluation for CHF, including an echocardiogram. If ascites is present (indicated by the positive fluid wave), liver function studies are needed. The edema associated with hypothyroidism would not cause ascites. A lower extremity Doppler evaluation would be indicated for unilateral edema. A urinalysis may be helpful in the setting of renal failure, but with ascites, liver tests would be more valuable.

184. The answer is b. *(Mengel, pp 132-136.)* In the workup of edema, the first thing to note is if the edema is bilateral or unilateral. Unilateral edema not associated with trauma or signs of infection requires a Doppler ultrasound to evaluate for the presence of DVT. The CT PE scan or the V̇/Q̇ scan would not be indicated unless there was suspicion of a PE.

185. The answer is e. *(Mengel, pp 132-136.)* Unilateral edema is suspicious for a DVT. However, if there is a history of recent trauma, or evidence of inflammation, a Doppler ultrasound is usually not necessary. Signs of inflammation including erythema point toward cellulitis as a diagnosis.

186. The answer is c. *(Mengel, pp 132-136.)* In patients with chronic venous insufficiency, knee-length elastic stockings can aid venous return. Additional treatment options include leg elevation throughout the day. Prolonged standing should be limited. Unilateral edema usually does not respond to diuresis, sodium restriction, or an ACE inhibitor. The case described above would be unlikely to be related to a DVT because of its chronic nature.

187. The answer is c. *(Mengel, pp 137-140.)* It is important to classify enuresis correctly, as treatment may vary depending on type. Enuresis is classified as primary if it has never followed a period of dryness. Enuresis that occurs after 6 months of dryness is classified as secondary enuresis. Enuresis is nocturnal if it only happens at night, and diurnal if it happens during the day and at night. There is no classification of "primary intentional enuresis."

188. The answer is a. *(Mengel, pp 137-140.)* While the cause of nocturnal enuresis is unknown, it is felt to be due to decreased production of nocturnal antidiuretic hormone. It is not likely due to deep sleep, though most enuretic patients do not spontaneously awaken after bed wetting. It is associated with a maturational delay, and statistically 25% of 5-year-olds are enuretic. The numbers decrease about 15% per year. Forty to fifty percent of bedwetters are female. Family history is very important. If one parent was enuretic, there is a 40% likelihood that the child will be. If both parents were bed wetters, there is a 70% risk that the child will be. Interestingly, the child will usually stop around the same time that the parent did. Very few patients have an organic cause.

189. The answer is b. *(Mengel, pp 137-140.)* Enuresis alarms have been shown to be the most effective treatment for nocturnal enuresis. Initial cure rates are high, and relapse rates are low. The alarms need to be used appropriately, with parental involvement in order to be effective. Frequent nighttime wakening may be effective, but compliance is a barrier to effectiveness. DDAVP can also be effective, but relapse rate is high once the medication is discontinued. Tricyclics have a lower initial cure rate and a high relapse rate.

They can also be lethal, if overdosed. Oxybutynin has a high relapse rate and has not been proven to be efficacious when compared with placebo.

190. The answer is a. *(Rakel, pp 838-840.)* In the child with monosymptomatic nocturnal enuresis, no further evaluation is needed, other than a thorough voiding history, physical examination, and urinalysis. X-rays of the lumbar and sacral spine are indicated if there is suspicion of spina bifida occulta, and renal ultrasound/VCUG are indicated if there are suspected anatomic abnormalities that would lead to enuresis.

191. The answer is a. *(Rakel, pp 838-840.)* Treatment for nocturnal enuresis should be first directed at treating constipation. It often coexists, and when constipation is treated, the situation improves dramatically. Motivational therapy should be considered for families not interested in pharmacologic therapy, but should never include consequences for wetting. The child has no control over wet nights, and should never be punished for a wet bed. DDAVP, a synthetic analog of vasopressin, works well in the form of a nasal spray or oral pill, but should not be the first measure tried. Imipramine is a tricyclic antidepressant with anticholenergic side effects, including urinary retention. It is useful, but not as an initial measure. Tolterodine is a treatment for overactive bladder, and has not been shown to be helpful for simple nocturnal enuresis.

192. The answer is a. *(Rakel, pp 838-840.)* Moisture-sensitive alarms can be a very successful behavioral treatment for nocturnal enuresis. The first drops of urine complete a circuit, activating an alarm that will wake the child (and the parents). The parents then help the child complete voiding in the toilet. Over time, a conditioned response develops, and the child awakens voluntarily with the sensation of a full bladder. There is no gender difference in success rates, and with appropriate use and parent involvement, success rates are between 70% and 90%. It may take weeks or months to be successful, and requires a sizeable commitment from the parents and child involved. The child should not take responsibility for this treatment, because without parental involvement, success rates drop.

193. The answer is a. *(South-Paul, pp 13-20.)* The growth chart raises concern for failure to thrive. While there are several definitions, concern should be raised when a child drops more than two percentile brackets on a growth curve and does not maintain at that area. In the United States, the vast majority of failure to thrive is secondary to inadequate nutrition and a thorough dietary history is most likely to reveal the cause. Albumin has a long half-life, and is a poor indicator of recent undernutrition. Prealbumin is decreased in acute inflammation and undernutrition, and is therefore insensitive. Organic disease, including hypothyroidism, is found in less than 10% of cases of failure to thrive. IgA levels are sensitive to undernutrition and would be decreased in failure to thrive.

194. The answer is d. *(South-Paul, pp 13-20.)* In a child with failure to thrive diarrhea and recurrent respiratory infections, cystic fibrosis must be considered, and a sweat chloride test should be ordered. The other tests may be indicated in the workup of failure to thrive, but only with a reasonable degree of clinical suspicion. With the history given, the most useful test would be the sweat chloride test.

195. The answer is a. *(South-Paul, pp 13-20.)* Children with familial short stature have a growth curve that shows simultaneous changes in height and weight. In failure to thrive and constitutional growth delay, weight decreases first, then height. In hypothyroidism, height velocity slows first and may plateau before weight changes. In breast-fed infants, weight decreases relative to peers after 4 to 6 months, but catches up after 12 months.

196. The answer is e. *(South-Paul, pp 13-20.)* Hospital admission is indicated for failure to thrive, in the face of hypotension and bradycardia. These are signs of severe malnutrition. Other interventions may be appropriate, but with vital sign abnormalities, it is important to admit the patient. Patients like this are generally not neglected, especially since he has been seen all along for well-child checks.

197. The answer is d. *(Wolff, pp 548-550.)* Mononucleosis is often mistaken for streptococcal pharyngitis. Both have symptoms of sore throat, fatigue, fever, and adenopathy. If patients with mononucleosis are given ampicillin (and other penicillin derivatives), they often develop the rash described above, sometimes confused as an allergic reaction to penicillin. The rash of scarlet fever is more confluent, and has a sandpaper-like texture.

198. The answer is c. *(Mengel, pp 147-152.)* The most common causes of fatigue in primary care include depression, life stress, chronic medical conditions, and medication reactions. Red flags for other causes include all of the symptoms listed in this question. Chronic fatigue syndrome can be associated with unrefreshing sleep, postexertional fatigue, difficulty with concentration, and headaches. It is usually not associated with weight loss, and if that sign is present, one should look for other causes for fatigue.

199. The answer is a. *(Mengel, pp 147-152.)* Depression is one of the most common diagnoses in patients presenting with fatigue, especially when denying weakness or hypersomnolence. Once the complaint is defined, the practitioner should screen for depression. Screening for sleep apnea, anemia, hypothyroidism, and pregnancy should occur if the depression screen is negative.

200. The answer is b. *(Mengel, pp 147-152.)* There are three general categories of fatigue: physiological, physical, and psychological. Physiological fatigue is generally due to overwork, lack of sleep, or a defined physical stress, such as pregnancy. Physical fatigue is due to infections, endocrine imbalances, anemia, cardiovascular diseases, and more concerning causes like cancer. Psychological fatigue is generally associated with stress, depression, anxiety, or adjustment reaction. While all types of fatigue can last for 6 months, the progressive nature of this patient's symptoms should lead one to look for a physical cause. Increased stress, overwork, and alcohol use generally do not point to a physical cause of stress.

201. The answer is d. *(Mengel, pp 147-152.)* The initial laboratory workup for an uncertain diagnosis of fatigue included a CBC, sedimentation rate, urinalysis, chemistry panel, thyroid testing, pregnancy testing (for women of childbearing age), and age/gender appropriate cancer screening. In a 55-year-old African American male, a prostate screen would be appropriate. Chest x-ray, ECG, HIV test, and a drug screen would be appropriate if the initial screen is negative.

202. The answer is e. *(Mengel, pp 174-178.)* Meckel diverticulum is the most common cause of significant GI bleeding in children. It is a congenital abnormality that occurs in about 2% of the population, with a male to female ratio of 2 to 1. It occurs about 2 ft from the ileocecal valve, and is usually about 2 in long. About 2% of cases have complications. These facts are often remembered as "the rule of 2s." Intussusception also occurs in this age group, but is usually painful. Anal fissures, colitis, and juvenile polyposis generally do not cause significant bleeding.

203. The answer is c. *(Mengel, pp 174-178.)* Upper endoscopy is the best diagnostic testing option in the setting of an acute upper GI bleed. It can localize the source of bleeding, potentially allow therapeutic intervention, and allow for tissue diagnosis when necessary. Gastric lavage is less useful, and a barium study might interfere with subsequent intervention. Red cell scans are better to locate bleeding sources in the lower GI tract, and angiography may miss slower bleeds.

204. The answer is d. *(Rakel, pp 617-621.)* Meckel diverticulum is the most common congenital abnormality of the GI tract, present in about 2% of the population. Most are asymptomatic, but a common presentation is painless large-volume intestinal hemorrhage. A Meckel diverticulum is often incidentally diagnosed at laparotomy. A noninvasive diagnostic modality is the technetium scan, often called the "Meckel scan." The labeled tracer is picked up by the heterotopic gastric mucosa in the diverticulum. A Meckel diverticulum is located in the distal ileum, and would not be identified by the other endoscopic procedures mentioned in the question.

205. The answer is c. *(Rakel, pp 617-621.)* Approximately 5% to 15% of patients with colonic diverticulosis develop severe diverticular bleeding. While many believe it may be triggered by the ingestion of certain foods, this has never been proven by studies. It is unusual to find the source of bleeding during colonoscopy. If colonoscopy does not localize the bleeding, a tagged RBC scan should be the next step, and will help guide segmental resection if necessary. A subtotal colectomy is only necessary for recurrent severe bleeding with no source identified.

206. The answer is e. *(Rakel, pp 639-643.)* The condition described is a thrombosed external hemorrhoid. External hemorrhoids are defined as hemorrhoids arising distal to the dentate line. When they thrombose, they are associated with acute pain and are hard and nodular on physical examination. The excision can be safely done in the office with local anesthesia. It eliminates pain immediately and eliminates the risk of reoccurrence. Hydrocortisone would not be helpful. Rubber band ligation and sclerotherapy should be reserved for internal hemorrhoids. Incision and drainage of the hemorrhoid increases the risk of reoccurrence and can lead to infection of the retained clot.

207. The answer is a. *(Rakel, pp 639-643.)* An anal fissure is a split in the anoderm of the anal canal. It generally occurs after the passage of a hard bowel movement. Patients present with excruciating pain on defecation with blood found on the toilet paper. After the bowel movement, the patient may complain of an ache or spasm that resolves after a couple of hours. Thrombosed external hemorrhoids would generally be visible on examination. Internal hemorrhoids are generally not painful, unless they are thrombosed because of an unreducible prolapse. If that were the case, the pain would not resolve. A perianal abscess may not present with bleeding, but would likely be associated with systemic signs of infection.

208. The answer is a. (*South-Paul, pp 289-297.*) While any and all of the choices listed as answers may be necessary in the initial evaluation of a headache, the most important way to characterize the headache is by history. Physical examination would be confirmatory. Blood work, imaging, and consultation may be important in the management, but only after the characterization of the headache as migraine, cluster, tension, or secondary headache.

209. The answer is a. (*South-Paul, pp 289-297.*) While many agents, including some anticonvulsants, have been used as prophylactic agents to prevent migraines, β-blockers are the most studied, and are effective. Verapamil is the only calcium channel blocker that studies show to have a prophylactic effect. There has been some interest in fluoxetine for prophylactic therapy, but more studies are needed. Ergotamines are used for abortive therapy.

210. The answer is a. (*South-Paul, pp 289-297*) The goal of prophylactic migraine therapy is to reduce the frequency of headache by 50%. Of the antidepressants, the strongest evidence for efficacy involves amitriptyline. Therapy begins with a low dose (10 mg at night) and can be titrated up to the most effective dose that does not cause prohibitive side effects (up to 150 mg). SSRIs, MAOIs, and other antidepressants have been variably studied, but the best evidence supports the use of amitriptyline, a tricyclic antidepressant.

211. The answer is a. (*South-Paul, pp 289-297*) Warning signs include a headache that has its onset after the age of 50 years, a very sudden onset, increase in severity or frequency, with signs of systemic disease, focal neurologic symptoms (except those consistent with a visual aura typical for a known migraine sufferer), papilledema, or a headache after trauma. Migraines often occur in a consistent location, are severe and frequent, include a visual aura, and may be associated with severe nausea.

212. The answer is e. *(McPhee, pp 837-841.)* Although frequently used in emergency settings, narcotics are rarely needed in the treatment plan for migraine sufferers. Simple analgesics, if taken early in the episode, often provide relief. Cafergot, an ergotamine plus caffeine, is often helpful. Because of impaired absorption and/or vomiting, rectal preparations can be used. Serotonin (5-HT) antagonists are rapidly effective.

213. The answer is b. *(South-Paul, pp 289-297.)* Verapamil appears to have some migraine prophylactic effect, but there is no evidence that other calcium channel blockers have a similar effect. Other calcium channel blockers may be helpful in suppressing cluster headaches, but have not been shown to be helpful for migraines.

214. The answer is d. *(South-Paul, pp 289-297.)* The mainstay of therapy for cluster headaches is to provide relief from the acute attacks, then use therapy to suppress headaches during the symptomatic period. Nifedipine has been shown to be effective, as has prednisone, indomethacin, and lithium. However, the medication should not be given daily, just during the symptomatic period. Fluoxetine has not been shown to be beneficial, and ergotamine is generally only helpful in the acute stage—not for prophylaxis.

215. The answer is e. *(McPhee, pp 837-841.)* Cluster headaches characteristically develop rapidly, achieving peak intensity within 10 to 15 minutes. Usually, the headaches are intensely painful and last for about 2 hours without treatment. The mainstay of treatment is oxygen. In general, oral medications are not helpful. Intravenous or intramuscular ergotamine has been shown to be helpful, as has injectable sumatriptan.

216. The answer is b. *(South-Paul, pp 289-297.)* Tension-type headaches (TTH) have a formal definition, with positive and negative criteria for diagnosis, but many physicians diagnose this type of headache by exclusion (after ruling out more interesting or rare etiologies for headache). They are in fact, the most frequent of all headaches encountered in clinical practice. The episodes last from 30 minutes to several days, and headaches should occur less than 15 times per month. It requires at least two of the following characteristics:

- Pressure/tightness
- Bilateral

- Mild to moderate
- Not aggravated by activity

There is generally no nausea. Either photophobia or phonophobia may be present, but not both. If criteria for this classification of headache are met, a trial of NSAIDs may be appropriate, with follow-up if there is no improvement. Narcotics should be avoided, since the condition is generally chronic, and overuse is likely. Imaging would not be helpful or indicated at this stage.

217. The answer is c. (*South-Paul, pp 289-297.*) Alarm symptoms for headaches should prompt the clinician to search for a secondary cause. These include new onset of headaches after the age of 50, very sudden onset, headaches that increase in severity or frequency, new onset headache in someone with risks for HIV or cancer, headache with signs of systemic illness, focal neurological symptoms, papilledema, or headache following head trauma. In these cases, further workup should be considered, and dictated by the differential diagnosis. In the patient described in this question, his age should raise the suspicion of temporal arteritis or mass lesion.

218. The answer is b. (*Mengel, pp 219-223.*) There are several medications that can cause hematuria. They include penicillins, cephalosporins, sulfonamides, phenytoin, cyclophosphamide, mitotane, anticoagulants, and nitrofurantoin. Ibuprofen may cause kidney problems, but hematuria is not one of them.

219. The answer is e. (*Mengel, pp 219-223.*) Painless hematuria without other symptoms is the most common presentation of bladder carcinoma. Risk factors include being male, smoking, and working in the printing/leather dye industries. Acute prostatitis and UTIs are usually associated with dysuria, fever, and urinary frequency and urgency. Chronic prostatitis is associated with urinary symptoms as well. Stones are associated with pain.

220. The answer is d. (*Mengel, pp 219-223.*) Pseudohematuria can be derived from chemical agents, foods, or vaginal bleeding. Common foods that cause this include beets, blackberries, and rhubarb. Medications that discolor the urine include chloroquine, metronidazole, phenytoin, rifampin, and sulfasalazine, among others.

221. The answer is a. (*Mengel, pp 219-223.*) Terminal hematuria suggests either a bladder neck or a prostatic urethral lesion. Hematuria occurring throughout micturition occurs with bladder or renal lesions. Urolithiasis is associated with pain, and although urethral trauma is associated with hematuria, it would occur throughout micturition.

222. The answer is e. *(Mengel, pp 219-223.)* In a pediatric patient with hematuria, red cell casts and an elevated creatinine, glomerulonephritis is possible. Poststreptococcal infection accounts for 50% of all cases of pediatric hematuria. The other tests described in the question would identify stones or tumors, but those are unlikely in this age group.

223. The answer is a. *(Mengel, pp 219-223.)* In patients younger than 40 years with hematuria, but a normal IV pyelogram and urine culture, periodic monitoring and reassurance is appropriate. In a patient older than 40 years, cystoscopy or renal biopsy would be appropriate. A post-streptococcal glomerulonephritis would be unlikely in this age group, and a renal biopsy would not be needed if the creatinine is normal.

224. The answer is c. *(Rakel, pp 648-655.)* Hepatitis A is the most commonly reported hepatitis virus, and does not lead to chronic infection. Fecal shedding of the virus occurs early, and is no longer an issue at the time of presentation. Infectiousness is highest during the prodrome, and actually decreases by the time jaundice develops. Relapses of hepatitis A are rare, but do occur. Fulminant liver disease occurs in less than 1% of patients.

225. The answer is b. *(Rakel, pp 648-655.)* Hepatitis B infection is clearly associated with an increased risk of developing hepatocellular carcinoma, and has been labeled as having oncogenic properties.

226. The answer is a. *(Rakel, pp 648-655.)* Transmission of hepatitis B may occur through the transfer of blood or body fluids, but can also occur perinatally (vertical transmission). If the virus is acquired early in life, the infection is silent, but up to 90% of those infected develop chronic disease. Those with a compromised immune system may also develop chronic disease easier than healthy patients. Healthy adults infected have spontaneous resolution more than 95% of the time. As with infection with hepatitis A, a small percentage of those infected will develop fulminant liver disease.

227. The answer is a. *(Rakel, pp 648-655.)* Identifying the correct stage of hepatitis B infection relies heavily on the correct interpretation of serologic markers. The first marker to appear after infection is usually HBsAg. It may appear prior to the onset of clinical symptoms, and usually disappears in a few weeks as the patient recovers. HBcAg is a protein contained in the inner core of the virion and is not found in the serum. The antibody to the core protein is found early, and persists indefinitely. The HBeAg correlates with active replication.

228. The answer is a. (*Rakel, pp 648-655.*) Unlike hepatitis B virus, the hepatitis C virus has not been found in body fluids other than blood, and the virus is primarily transmitted through exposure to blood and blood products.

229. The answer is c. (*Rakel, pp 648-655.*) The HBsAg positivity in this case indicates either chronic infection or early infection. The negativity of the IgM anti-HBc rules out an early infection. The HBeAg is correlated with replication, as is the HBV-DNA.

230. The answer is e. (*Rakel, pp 648-655.*) The positivity of the anti-HBs indicates either exposure with immunity, recovery phase, or vaccination. Because the IgG anti-HBc is negative, there is no evidence of past exposure or infection.

231. The answer is a. (*Rakel, pp 648-655.*) The HBsAg positivity in this case indicates either chronic infection or early infection. The positivity of the IgM anti-HBc indicates early infection, and is negative in chronic infection. If the patient were in the recovery phase, his HBsAg would be negative.

232. The answer is b. (*South-Paul, pp 462-472.*) Contrary to common perception, urinary incontinence is not inevitable with aging. However, many common age-related changes do predispose elderly patients to incontinence. It is important to remember that these changes are found in many healthy, continent elderly persons. Involuntary bladder contractions increase with age, potentially leading to urge incontinence. Total bladder contractility decreases with age, potentially leading to overflow incontinence. Elderly patients excrete a larger percentage of fluid late in the day (increasing nocturia), and urogenital atrophy leads to decreased internal urethral sphincter sensitivity, potentially leading to stress incontinence.

233. The answer is d. (*South-Paul, pp 462-472.*) Asymptomatic bacteriuria is common in otherwise well elderly, and does not cause incontinence—whereas, a symptomatic infection may. Hyperglycemia can cause secondary incontinence because of polyuria, and continence can be restored by more tightly controlling the patient's sugar. Diuretics also may cause secondary incontinence, and may need to be avoided unless necessary. Stool impaction is thought to be a causative factor in up to 10% of patients with incontinence, and disimpaction may restore continence. Atrophic vaginitis may also be causative, and treatment may improve the situation.

234. The answer is c. (*South-Paul, pp 462-472.*) Urge incontinence is the most common type of incontinence in the elderly. Due to detrusor hyperactivity, patients often complain of a strong urge followed by an involuntary loss of urine. Functional incontinence refers to a limitation that does not allow the patient to void in the bathroom (bed rest, paralysis, severe dementia) and does not generally relate to the urinary tract. Stress incontinence is the loss of urine associated with increased intra-abdominal pressure, and overflow incontinence is due to overdistention of the bladder. Senile incontinence is a fictional term.

235. The answer is d. (*South-Paul, pp 462-472.*) Stress incontinence is much more commonly seen in women than in men, and is most often caused by urethral hypermobility resulting from weakness of the pelvic floor musculature. Patients complain of involuntary loss of urine associated with increase in intra-abdominal pressure (when sneezing, coughing, laughing, or exercising). Functional incontinence refers to a limitation that does not allow the patient to void in the bathroom (bed rest, paralysis, severe dementia) and does not generally relate to the urinary tract. Urge incontinence is the loss of urine following a strong urge, and overflow incontinence is due to overdistention of the bladder. Senile incontinence is a fictional term.

236. The answer is e. (*South-Paul, pp 462-472.*) Overflow incontinence is primarily a loss of the ability to empty the bladder, usually due to neurogenic bladder (longstanding diabetes, alcoholism, disk disease) or because of outlet obstruction (prostatic enlargement). In this case, the patient usually complains of a frequent or constant leakage of small amount, but occasionally a large amount of urine is lost without warning. Functional incontinence refers to a limitation that does not allow the patient to void in the bathroom (bed rest, paralysis, severe dementia) and does not generally relate to the urinary tract. Stress incontinence is the loss of urine associated with increased abdominal pressure, and urge incontinence is preceded by a strong urge to urinate. Senile incontinence is a fictional term.

237. The answer is e. (*South-Paul, pp 462-472.*) After ruling out secondary causes of incontinence, a postvoid residual measurement should be taken. This can be done through catheterization or via ultrasound. A postvoid residual less than 50 mL is normal. A postvoid residual greater than 200 mL indicates inadequate bladder emptying and is consistent with overflow incontinence. Between 50 and 200 mL is indeterminate.

238. The answer is b. (*South-Paul, pp 462-472.*) Kegel exercises are designed to strengthen the pelvic floor musculature. Patients are asked to squeeze the muscles in the genital area as if they were trying to stop the flow of urine from the urethra. They hold this contraction for 10 seconds, and repeat this many times in the day. Patients are then taught to contract these muscles and hold them during situations where incontinence may occur. They are most useful to treat stress incontinence, but may help with mixed incontinence as well. It is not helpful for functional, urge, or overflow incontinence.

239. The answer is a. (*South-Paul, pp 462-472.*) Pharmacological therapy is indicated for incontinence if a behavioral approach is ineffective. For urge incontinence, anticholinergic medications are the drugs of choice with oxybutynin (Ditropan) and tolterodine (Detrol) both indicated for symptoms. Pseudoephedrine has been shown to help stress incontinence, trimethoprim-sulfamethoxazole has been shown to help in the case of prostatitis, and finasteride and terazosin will help frequent voiding caused by prostatic hyperplasia.

240. The answer is c. (*South-Paul, pp 462-272.*) Pharmaceuticals are a common cause of incontinence. There are many neural receptors involved in urination, and therefore many medications use to treat other medical issues can often cause problems. Antihypertensives are especially problematic. α-Blockers cause urethral sphincter relaxation and can cause urinary leakage, but not urgency. Calcium channel blockers can cause urinary retention. Diuretics can cause increased frequency and urgency, but usually not leakage. β-Blockers inhibit bladder relaxation and therefore can cause both urinary leakage and urgency.

241. The answer is e. (*South-Paul, pp 462-472.*) Many nonprescription agents may contribute to urinary symptoms. Alcohol has a diuretic effect and may cause polyuria or incontinence. Decongestants and diet pills may cause urinary retention if they include α-agonists. Antihistamines can cause urinary retention or functional incontinence. Caffeine has a diuretic effect, and can cause polyuria. Marijuana abuse is not known to contribute to urinary symptoms.

242. The answer is a. (*South-Paul, pp 133-145.*) Primary amenorrhea is defined as the absence of menses at age 16 in the presence of normal secondary sex characteristics, or absence of menses at age 14 in the absence of secondary sex characteristics. It is usually the result of a genetic or anatomic abnormality. Gonadal dysgenesis is the most common cause of primary amenorrhea, responsible for about 50% of the cases. The most well-known type is Turner syndrome (45 XO). Hypothalamic failure is often a result of anorexia nervosa, excessive exercise, chronic or systemic illness, and severe stress, and results from a suppression of hypothalamic gonadotropin-releasing hormone (GnRH) secretion. Pituitary failure may result from inadequate GnRH stimulation and is often associated with a history of head trauma, shock, infiltrative processes, pituitary adenoma, or craniopharyngioma. These patients will often display deficiency of other pituitary hormones as well. Polycystic ovarian syndrome may cause primary amenorrhea, but is generally associated with normal breast development. Constitutional delay of puberty, although common in boys, is an uncommon cause of amenorrhea in girls, but clinically is very hard to distinguish from other more common causes.

243. The answer is c. (*South-Paul, pp 133-145.*) Pregnancy is the most common cause of secondary amenorrhea, and can even occur in a patient who claims that she has not been sexually active or says that she only has intercourse during "safe" times. Polycystic ovarian syndrome is common, and is responsible for about 30% of the cases of secondary amenorrhea. It is characterized by androgen excess, and symptoms include irregular or absent menses, hirsutism, acne, and virilization. Functional hypothalamic amenorrhea is usually a result of anorexia, rapid weight loss, rigorous exercise, or significant emotional stress. Hypothyroidism and hyperprolactinemia can both be associated with secondary amenorrhea, but are less common causes.

244. The answer is c. (*South-Paul, pp 133-145. Mengel, pp 387-391.*) Anovulatory bleeding is caused by continuous unopposed endometrial estrogen stimulation. Since these patients do not ovulate, progesterone from the corpus luteum is not secreted, the withdrawal from which would normally cause endometrial sloughing. It is the most common cause of dysfunctional uterine bleeding in women younger than 20 years of age, accounting for about 95% of cases. When women are within 2 years of menarche, this is especially common, and can be followed expectantly. Alternatively, oral contraceptives can be used to regulate periods. Pregnancy should be ruled out, even in women who deny sexual activity. Ovulatory bleeding due to fluctuations in estrogen and progesterone levels is also a cause of abnormal bleeding, but accounts for only about 10% of cases. Leiomyomas and polyps may cause bleeding, but usually not in this age group.

245. The answer is d. (*Mengel, pp 387-391.*) If a postmenopausal woman has vaginal bleeding, she needs an endometrial biopsy to rule out endometrial cancer. In fact, this is usually the first step in the evaluation of this problem, after performing the examination and ruling out sexually transmitted infections or anatomic abnormalities. Ultrasound evaluation may be needed, but this would not be the next step in the evaluation of this condition. Contraindications to this procedure include pregnancy, acute infection, PID, or known bleeding disorder (including Coumadin use).

246. The answer is a. (*South-Paul, pp 133-145.*) Primary dysmenorrhea is caused by the release of prostaglandin from the endometrium at the time of menstruation. Treatment focuses on the reduction of endometrial prostaglandin production. This can occur either by using medications that inhibit prostaglandin synthesis, or by suppressing ovulation. NSAIDs are generally the first line of therapy, given their favorable risk to benefit ratio and effectiveness. They should be started a day before menstruation, if possible. Daily use of NSAIDs does not increase effectiveness, and is associated with an increase of side effects. While opiate use may help with pain control, it does not inhibit prostaglandin synthesis and may lead to addiction. SSRI therapy is sometimes used for premenstrual dysphoric disorder, but is not a first-line therapy for dysmenorrhea. Oral contraceptive pills can be used and are effective, but are thought of as second-line therapy.

247. The answer is a. (*Mengel, pp 13-17.*) Turner syndrome is the most common karyotypic abnormality associated with amenorrhea. It is associated with short stature, a webbed neck, and sexual infantilism. Fragile X and Down syndrome are associated with developmental delay, but not necessarily short stature. Testicular feminization would be associated with amenorrhea, but not with the physical examination findings of Turner syndrome. Factor V Leiden deficiency would not be associated with amenorrhea.

248. The answer is b. (*Mengel, pp 13-17.*) Many medications can cause hyperprolactinemia leading to amenorrhea. When hyperprolactinemia is related to medication, the measured prolactin level is usually less than 100 ng/mL. Many psychotropic medications can cause this, including benzodiazepines, SSRIs, tricyclic antidepressants, phenothiazines, and buspirone. Neurologic drugs that can increase prolactin levels include sumatriptan, valproate, and ergot derivatives. Estrogens and contraceptives can also elevate prolactin, as can some cardiovascular drugs (atenolol, verapamil, reserpine, and methyldopa). This is a less likely side effect in proton pump inhibitors, diuretics, ACE inhibitors, and thyroid replacement.

249. The answer is e. (*Mengel, pp 13-17.*) The progestin challenge test separates patients with estrogen deficiency from those with normal or excess estrogen. Any bleeding in the week after the administration of Provera indicates that the patient has sufficient estrogen to menstruate, and that the amenorrhea is likely due to anovulation, as in polycystic ovarian syndrome. Those with premature ovarian failure would not have a withdrawal bleed. Neoplasm, Turner syndrome, and Asherman syndrome would not likely present in this way.

250. The answer is a. (*Mengel, pp 13-17.*) Patients with amenorrhea and elevated testosterone and DHEA-S levels need CT scanning of the adrenal glands and ultrasound of the ovaries to rule out neoplasm. Hysteroscopy and hysterosalpingogram may be involved in the workup of menstrual irregularities or infertility, but would not be helpful in the setting of hormonal abnormalities described. MRI would be helpful if pituitary tumor were suspected, and karyotyping would be appropriate to rule out genetic abnormalities, neither of which is suspected in this case.

251. The answer is a. (*Mengel, pp 13-17.*) When evaluating primary amenorrhea in patients with normal secondary sexual characteristics and a normal initial laboratory evaluation (pregnancy test, TSH assessment, and prolactin level), it is appropriate to perform a progestin challenge test. When there is no withdrawal bleeding, it either indicates inadequate estrogen production or an outflow tract obstruction. An estrogen-progestin challenge can differentiate between the two. No withdrawal bleeding after an estrogen-progestin challenge indicates an outflow tract obstruction or an anatomic defect.

252. The answer is a. (*Mengel, pp 13-17.*) Primary dysmenorrhea is defined as pain with menstruation, not associated with identified pelvic pathology.

Secondary dysmenorrhea is associated with identified pelvic pathology. In general, if the history and physical examination are normal, no further workup is necessary, and a trial of treatment is indicated. Gonorrhea and *Chlamydia* cultures may be necessary in the initial evaluation, but if the history and examination are not suggestive of infection, cultures are not necessary. Ultrasound, hysterosalpingography, and laparoscopy are not indicated at this stage of the evaluation.

253. The answer is b. *(Mengel, pp 108-112.)* The history described is classic for primary dysmenorrhea. Oral contraceptive pills are an appropriate choice for treatment. They work by suppressing menstrual fluid volume and prostaglandin release, but not synthesis. This is achieved through endometrial hypoplasia. NSAIDs decrease prostaglandin production. Oral contraceptives do not increase vasoconstriction of the uterus or directly impact uterine tone.

254. The answer is a. *(Mengel, pp 60-66.)* Delirium and dementia are often clinically difficult to distinguish, especially if you are unfamiliar with the patient. Disorientation is characteristic of both processes, as is a disturbed sleep-wake cycle. His history of hypertension would lead one to think of multi-infarct dementia, rather than delirium. Responsiveness to questions may be a feature of either process, though patients with delirium often have a shortened attention span. The abrupt onset of a mental status change is consistent with delirium as opposed to dementia, which occurs insidiously.

255. The answer is c. *(Mengel, pp 60-66.)* The patient described has a hypertensive encephalopathy. With his severe hypertension, a stroke may be considered, but unlikely without focal neurological deficits. Sixth nerve palsy may be seen in a stroke. Pinpoint pupils would be more consistent with narcotic excess, unlikely given his vital signs and history. Dilated pupils suggests sympathetic outflow, and may be consistent with delirium tremens, but the history and physical is not consistent with this. Papilledema is seen with hypertensive encephalopathy. Anisocoria of 1 mm is a nonspecific finding that can be seen in normal individuals.

256. The answer is d. *(Mengel, pp 60-66.)* Hyperalert confusion is common with alcohol withdrawal. Hypothyroidism would present with fatigue and psychomotor slowing. Fluoxetine usually does not cause a withdrawal syndrome, but may be associated with depressive symptoms. Opiate withdrawal does not present with a confusional state. Amphetamine withdrawal would be associated with psychomotor slowing.

257. The answer is e. *(Mengel, pp 60-66.)* While a urinalysis, CBC, toxicology screen, and pregnancy test may all reveal the cause of delirium, the patient's history is consistent with viral or bacterial meningitis. A lumbar puncture is the most likely test to reveal the diagnosis in this case.

258. The answer is c. *(Mengel, pp 60-66.)* In dementia, the level of consciousness is not clouded, but disorientation may occur later in the illness. Hypertension and diabetes may be seen with both delirium and dementia. The inability to complete serial sevens (count backward from 100 by 7s) may be related to educational level. Although his symptoms have appeared recently, it is often difficult to pinpoint the exact onset of dementia. Delirium is seen as being more abrupt in onset.

259. The answer is c. *(Rakel, pp 5-10.)* While all of the medications listed have antiemetic properties, the patient described has gastroparesis, likely as a result of her longstanding diabetes. Metoclopramide can improve gastric motility and help her symptoms more than the other antiemetics listed.

260. The answer is c. *(Rakel, pp 5-10.)* A careful history and physical examination can often distinguish between potential causes for nausea and vomiting. In this case, mild pain, followed by the acute onset of distension, nausea, and vomiting is consistent with ileus or obstruction. Hyperactive bowel sounds lead one to think of obstruction; with an ileus bowel sounds are absent. Gastroenteritis begins acutely, but is usually not preceded by mild abdominal pain. Diverticulosis and diverticulitis would cause pain, but would be less likely to present with nausea, vomiting, and distension.

261. The answer is b. *(Rakel, pp 5-10.)* Psychogenic vomiting should be suspected in patients who are able to maintain adequate nutrition despite chronic symptoms. It is usually seen during times of social stress or in patients with a past history of a psychiatric disorder. Chronic gastroenteritis is an unlikely condition. While young girls in this age group are at risk for anorexia and bulimia, sufferers usually do not seek medical attention or treatment until concerned others bring the condition to medical attention. A central nervous system malignancy is possible, if the lesion involves the vomiting center, but one would expect to see nutritional deficit in that case.

262. The answer is b. *(Rakel, pp 5-10.)* The situation described is consistent with viral gastroenteritis, a common clinical condition. The Norwalk virus, reoviruses, and adenoviruses are common causes. Symptoms typically begin acutely and are associated with typical viral syndrome symptoms. Generally, these illnesses are self-limited, and will resolve within 5 days. Oral rehydration is indicated as long as there are no signs of severe dehydration. IV rehydration and antiemetics may have a role, but only in more severe cases. There is no role for antibiotic therapy.

263. The answer is d. *(Rakel, pp 5-10.)* The patient described has pancreatitis, likely due to gallstones. While the laboratory findings in acute pancreatitis are often nonspecific, elevated serum amylase in the right clinical setting is often suggestive. Radiographic evidence can help confirm the diagnosis. In establishing a cause for pancreatitis, history is key, but some laboratory findings are helpful. Elevated ALT is more suggestive of gallstone pancreatitis, and is less likely when alcohol or hypertriglyceridemia is the cause. ACE inhibitors are an uncommon cause of pancreatitis. Hypercalcemia is also a rare cause, but is unlikely in this case.

264. The answer is e. *(Mengel, pp 288-295.)* The symptoms and characteristics of nausea and vomiting can often be clues to the etiology. When nausea happens before eating in the morning, likely etiologies include pregnancy, uremia, alcohol withdrawal, and increased intracranial pressure (meningitis or space-occupying lesions). Gastroparesis and pancreatitis is usually associated with nausea after eating. Cholelithiasis is associated with nausea, vomiting, and pain after eating fatty foods. Vestibular disorders cause nausea without any clear association with meals or time of day.

265. The answer is a. *(Mengel, pp 288-295.)* Gastroparesis is associated with nausea and vomiting delayed 1 hour or more after eating. The vomit is nonbilious and the food is undigested. In the face of obesity, this may be secondary to undiagnosed and untreated type 2 diabetes. Nausea associated with cholelithiasis is associated with pain, usually after eating fatty foods. The nausea from pancreatitis is usually after meals, and is associated with pain. Vestibular disorders cause nausea without clear relationship to eating, and a brain tumor would cause morning symptoms.

266. The answer is c. *(Mengel, pp 288-295.)* Children with pyloric stenosis usually present with weight loss, dehydration, and occasionally a palpable "olive" mass in the epigastric area. It usually is identified before 7 weeks of age. Breast milk allergies are uncommon. Reflux may be possible, but is less likely to be associated with weight loss and dehydration. Intussusception is associated with significant abdominal pain, and hemoccult positive stools. Small-bowel obstruction is less likely, and would be associated with high-pitched bowel sounds.

267. The answer is b. (*Mengel, pp 288-295.*) Pancreatitis is associated with the acute onset of significant nausea, vomiting, and epigastric pain. The symptoms occur after eating, and are improved when the patient does not eat. Amylase and lipase are likely to be abnormal, but the CBC is likely to be normal. Hemoccult testing, abdominal x-rays, and upper endoscopy are likely to be normal.

268. The answer is d. (*Mengel, pp 288-295.*) The patient described likely has cholelithiasis. Nausea, vomiting, and pain occur after eating fatty meals. The diagnostic test of choice would be a right upper quadrant ultrasound to identify stones in the gallbladder. Amylase and lipase may be positive if the patient develops secondary pancreatitis, but are unlikely to be elevated until that point. Hemoccult testing, abdominal x-rays, and upper endoscopy are all likely to be normal.

269. The answer is d. (*Mengel, pp 288-295.*) Antiemetics can cause a variety of side effects. The phenothiazines (Compazine and Phenergan) generally cause drowsiness, dry mouth, and dizziness. Tigan causes similar side effects. Zofran is a serotonin receptor antagonist, and may cause dizziness and headache. Reglan is a prokinetic agent, and can cause diarrhea and extrapyramidal reactions.

270. The answer is c. (*Mengel, pp 300-306.*) There are several characteristics of palpitations that can help the physician determine whether or not the symptoms are from a cardiac cause. These include male sex, the description of the symptom as an "irregular heartbeat," a personal history of heart disease, and event duration greater than 5 minutes. Family history of similar symptoms would not be a risk factor for cardiac disease.

271. The answer is a. (*Mengel, pp 300-306.*) When a patient describes her heartbeat as rapid and irregular, it suggests either atrial fibrillation or atrial flutter. Ectopy and atrial fibrillation can both cause an irregular pulse. PSVT is usually rapid and regular, as is stable ventricular tachycardia. Stimulant abuse will generally cause a sinus tachycardia. While hyperthyroidism may cause atrial fibrillation, the patient would likely have additional symptoms.

272. The answer is c. (*Mengel, pp 300-306.*) Ventricular premature beats are often random, episodic, and instantaneous beats, often described as a "flip-flopping" sensation. Atrial fibrillation is described more as a rapid and irregular heart rate or a "fluttering" in the chest. PSVT is generally rapid and regular, and lasting a longer time. Stimulant abuse would likely cause sinus tachycardia, and while hyperthyroidism can cause premature beats, the patient would likely experience other symptoms.

273. The answer is b. (*Mengel, pp 300-306.*) Hypertrophic cardiomyopathy can be associated with atrial fibrillation or ventricular tachycardia. The characteristic heart murmur associated with it is a systolic ejection murmur (like aortic stenosis) worsening with Valsalva maneuver. Mitral valve prolapse would have a different characteristic murmur. Dilated cardiomyopathy and CHF would likely be associated with other symptoms. Atrial fibrillation would not be associated with a regular rhythm.

274. The answer is a. (*Mengel, pp 300-306.*) When the history, physical examination, 12-lead ECG, and limited laboratory evaluation are negative, it is appropriate to reassure the patient with palpitations and continue observation. The likely etiology is benign supraventricular or ventricular ectopy. Other tests and consultation would only be indicated if the patient's symptoms are incapacitating or worrisome.

275. The answer is d. (*Mengel, pp 300-306.*) Since this patient's arrhythmia only seems to occur with exercise, stress testing would be useful. Ambulatory ECG monitoring and echocardiography would not be useful. Consultation with an electrophysiologist may be appropriate, depending on the results of the testing.

276. The answer is c. (*Mengel, pp 300-306.*) The classic Wolff-Parkinson-White syndrome (preexcitation syndrome) ECG demonstrates a short PR interval and δ-waves. Patients are treated if they have symptomatic arrhythmia. Treatment usually consists of radiofrequency ablation, but pharmacologic therapy is also an option.

277. The answer is c. (*Mengel, pp 313-320.*) Classically, ovarian cysts present with a unilateral dull pain that can become diffuse and severe if the cyst ruptures. On physical examination, the examiner feels a smooth mobile adnexal mass with peritoneal signs if the cyst ruptures. PID is associated with fever and vaginal discharge. Ectopic pregnancy may present with similar symptoms, but menses would not be normal. Uterine leiomyoma would be associated with an enlarged uterus, and appendicitis would be associated with nausea and anorexia.

278. The answer is a. (*Mengel, pp 313-320.*) PID is classically described as lower abdominal pain that is gradual in onset and bilateral. Fever, vaginal discharge, dysuria, and occasionally abnormal vaginal bleeding may be associated symptoms. The minimal diagnostic criteria include uterine, adnexal, or cervical motion tenderness. Treatment should provide coverage for likely etiologic agents (*Neisseria gonorrhoeae, Chlamydia trachomatis,* anaerobes, and enteric gram-negative rods).

279. The answer is b. (*Mengel, pp 313-320.*) The pain associated with ectopic pregnancy is often described as colicky, and may radiate to the shoulder if there is a significant hemoperitoneum. Amenorrhea and symptoms of pregnancy are diagnostic clues.

280. The answer is e. (*Mengel, pp 313-320.*) The patient described has symptoms and signs suggestive of endometriosis. A CBC would be helpful if the signs are suggestive of an infectious process (appendicitis or PID). An ESR is elevated in 75% of patients with PID, but is nonspecific. CA-125 levels may be helpful if the physician is concerned about an ovarian mass. Transvaginal ultrasound may be helpful, but MRI is more sensitive for localization of endometriosis.

281. The answer is c. (*Mengel, pp 313-320.*) Eighty percent of ovarian masses in girls younger than 15 years are malignant. Because of the high potential for malignancy, any adnexal mass should be evaluated by transvaginal ultrasound and referral for surgical removal. In many women of childbearing years, adnexal masses are commonly cysts. If the pain is not acute or recurrent, palpable cysts less than 6 cm in size may be monitored with repeat pelvic examination. Ultrasound is reserved for those masses that do not resolve, or those that increase in size. CT and MRI may be useful in some cases, but the ultrasound is the best first test.

282. The answer is e. *(Rakel, pp 268-272.)* Any of the conditions listed as answers in this question can cause an exudative pharyngitis. Palatal petechiae suggest either a group A streptococcal infection of EBV pharyngitis. However, posterior cervical adenopathy should point to EBV as the correct diagnosis.

283. The answer is d. *(Rakel, pp 268-272.)* Fever, chills, myalgias, and pain with swallowing are nonspecific signs, and are associated with pharyngitis from any cause. Anterior adenopathy is also associated with viral or bacterial pharyngitis. However, uveal edema is suggestive of group A hemolytic streptococcal infection. First-line treatment should be amoxicillin, as up to 15% of group A streptococcal infections are resistant to penicillin. Doxycycline can be a good second-line agent. Macrolides are not generally effective, as they have poor penetration and may induce resistance.

284. The answer is b. *(Rakel, pp 268-272.)* Approximately 30% of patients with infectious mononucleosis are colonized with group A streptococcal organisms. Therefore, their rapid streptococcal antigen and throat cultures may be positive. When patients with mononucleosis are treated with penicillin or amoxicillin, they often develop a maculopapular skin rash that may be confused with scarlet fever. This should not be considered an allergic reaction. The distinguishing feature in this case is posterior chain adenopathy, consistent with an infectious mononucleosis.

285. The answer is e. *(Rakel, pp 268-272.)* The best antibiotics to eliminate group A streptococcal carriage from oropharyngeal secretions are an oral respiratory quinolone or oral clindamycin. The other therapies would be less likely to eliminate colonization.

286. The answer is a. *(Rakel, pp 268-272.)* Laryngitis with pharyngitis is generally associated with a viral infection, and only supportive care is needed. Antibiotic therapy is not indicated in this case.

287. The answer is d. *(McPhee, pp 191-192)* The clinical features most suggestive of group A β-hemolytic streptococcal pharyngitis are fever, tender anterior cervical adenopathy, lack of cough, and a pharyngotonsillar exudates.

These four features are called the Centor criteria, and when present, strongly ← 🖋
suggest infection, and the most cost effective approach is to treat without performing laboratory testing. When three of the four criteria are present, the
laboratory sensitivity of a rapid antigen test exceeds 90%. When only one cri-
terion is present, strep is unlikely. Marked adenopathy and a shaggy white-
purple tonsillar exudates is more suggestive of mononucleosis.

288. The answer is a. *(Rakel, pp 947-949.)* Acne is associated with many
myths regarding its cause. The true cause is multifactorial, but likely related
to disturbances of keratinization, hormonal secretion, and immune
response. Acne is not caused by dirt, diet, or oily hair on the forehead. Interestingly stress does likely play a role, but even then, just a small role.

289. The answer is b. *(Rakel, pp 947-949.)* The central lesion in acne is the
microcomedo. Therefore most acne treatment plans should involve a kera-
tolytic. Retinoids are excellent keratolytics, and may be used as monotherapy
in many cases, with the patients understanding that resolution may take
months. Topical erythromycin and clindamycin have become less useful as
monotherapy, as there has been a dramatic increase in resistance of *P acnes* to
the antibiotics alone. The addition of benzoyl peroxide to the regimen effectively prevents resistance. Oral antibiotics may work, but cephalosporins
should not be used. The medications of choice include erythromycins, tetracyclines trimethoprim-sulfamethoxazole, and ciprofloxacin. Oral contraceptives can often be used as an adjunct treatment in women, but most people
would not use it as a first-line agent. Topical steroids can be occasionally helpful, but invariably cause atrophy of the facial skin if used for too long. An
antibacterial cleanser would not be expected to be helpful alone.

290. The answer is b. *(Rakel, pp 947-949.)* Worsening acne in its most
severe form is acne fulminans. It must be avoided, as it leads to significant
scarring. Many families have heard that depression is a significant side effect
of isotretinoin, but large studies have failed to note any correlation. Dry skin
and joint aches are side effects, but shouldn't warrant discontinuing the medication unless intolerable. Pregnancy is not a side effect of medication, but if
it were to occur during the treatment, it would warrant discontinuation. Because
of the teratogenicity associated with isotretinoin, women taking the medication must use two forms of birth control—one hormonal and one barrier.
A pregnancy test must be obtained monthly, and treatment continued only if
it is negative.

291. The answer is b. (*Rakel, pp 947-949.*) The patient in the picture has rosacea. Although it is often considered along with acne, rosacea is a distinct entity. Comedo formation, the hallmark of acne vulgaris, is absent in rosacea. About 50% of the patients with rosacea have eye involvement, including styes, blepharitis, and corneal surface disease. Topical steroids should be avoided, as they ultimately make the disease worse. Oral tetracyclines are useful—isotretinoin is the last resort. Treatments aimed at reducing the colonization of *P acnes* without an anti-inflammatory treatment arm are not effective.

292. The answer is c. (*Rakel, pp 953-962.*) The patient shown has a classic nodular basal cell carcinoma, the most common type of basal cell cancer. It is characterized as a shiny papule, generally with a depressed central keratotic plug and visible telangiectasia near the border. Verruca do not generally have the depressed center or the pearly borders. Molluscum can look similar, but usually do not have the visible telangiectasia present. Squamous cell cancers generally have a scale and the absence of classic basal cell carcinoma (BCC) features. Cutaneous T-cell lymphoma have a variable presentation, usually with patches, plaques or tumors, and would be difficult to diagnosis by inspection alone.

293. The answer is e. (*Rakel, pp 962-970.*) The patient pictured has psoriasis. Topical corticosteroids are the most common therapeutic agents used to treat psoriasis. There is no place for antibiotics in treatment, except in the case of guttate psoriasis, a form that follows streptococcal infection and appears as multiple teardrops that erupt abruptly. Elidel is used for eczema, and although some use it to treat psoriasis, it is currently an off-label use. While the topical retinoid tazarotene (Tazorac) can be used, vitamin A is not indicated.

294. The answer is a. (*Rakel, pp 962-970.*) The rash shown is classic for pityriasis rosea, a self-limited papulosquamous eruption. The treatment includes antihistamines or corticosteroids to relieve itch. There is no role for the other agents listed.

295. The answer is b. (*Rakel, pp 1006-1010.*) The child shown has impetigo. This diagnosis should be considered in the face of well-demarcated erythematous lesions that, when disrupted, develop a secondary golden crust. The lesions have a predilection for traumatized skin, in this case where nasal discharge has disrupted the skin surface. In the past, most cases were thought to be due to streptococci. However, most cases are caused by *S aureus*.

296. The answer is a. *(Rakel, pp 1006-1010.)* The patient described and shown has "hot tub folliculitis." The infection is generally caused by *Pseudomonas aeruginosa* or *Pseudomonas cepacia*. However, the condition is usually self-limited. Antibiotic therapy is not indicated, except in recalcitrant cases, and usually reassurance is all that is necessary.

297. The answer is d. *(Rakel, pp 1010-1017.)* The description and picture are consistent with a recurrence of HSV infection. Symptomatic primary infections are characterized by gingivostomatitis with or without cutaneous or perioral lesions. Fever, malaise, and tender adenopathy are common with primary infections. Recurrences are usually less severe. The episode shown above is a recurrence because it appears as grouped vesicles as opposed to gingivostomatitis. There is no way to differentiate HSV-1 from HSV-2 simply by looking at the lesions. Lesions are sometimes mistaken for bacterial processes because they can be pustular. Triggers for recurrences are ultraviolet light exposure or illness.

298. The answer is e. *(South-Paul, pp 146-164.)* Treatment options for genital herpes include treating each outbreak (episodic therapy) or using chronic antiviral therapy on a daily basis to prevent outbreaks (suppressive therapy). If episodic therapy is used, it should begin at the first sign of an outbreak, but in discordant couples, daily suppressive therapy is now recommended. Suppressive therapy seems to reduce, not eliminate, asymptomatic viral shedding. Suppressive therapy does not alter the natural course of the infection, and is not associated with antiviral resistance. Daily suppressive therapy may reduce the risk of HIV transmission or acquisition, but more studies are needed.

299. The answer is b. *(Rakel, pp 1010-1017.)* The patient shown has herpes zoster, or "shingles." Antiviral therapy is the treatment of choice, and can decrease the time for lesion healing and shorten the overall duration of pain if initiated within 72 hours after the onset. In some cases, no benefit will occur if treatment starts after the 72 hour cutoff, but it should be initiated regardless of time in patients over 50, those who are immunosuppressed, or those with eye involvement. Corticosteroids have not been shown to decrease the likelihood of postherpetic neuralgia. No antiviral is clearly superior to another. Antiviral resistance is actually uncommon in this setting.

300. The answer is b. (*Rakel, pp 1010-1017.*) The picture shown, coupled with the clinical scenario described, is classic for infection with parvovirus B19. The resulting illness is called erythema infectiosum, or "fifth disease." Enteroviruses may cause hand-foot-and-mouth disease. Parainfluenza viruses are implicated in croup. Varicella causes chicken pox, and cytomegalovirus may cause mono-like symptoms, but not the classic "slapped cheek" appearing rash.

301. The answer is d. (*Rakel, pp 1021-1025.*) The picture shows tinea capitis. Systemic therapy is necessary for a cure, but concurrent use of topical ketoconazole shampoo or selenium sulfide lotion may kill spores on the hair. Griseofulvin is FDA approved for this indication, but fluconazole is not.

302. The answer is c. (*Rakel, pp 1021-1025.*) Tinea corporis, otherwise called "ringworm" is usually caused by *Trichophyton rubrum*. It appears as a well-demarcated plaque with central scaling. It is usually pruritic. Pityriasis rosea begins with a herald patch and develops as finer diffuse lesions. Psoriasis is generally found on the extensor surfaces of the skin, and would be unlikely to appear for the first time in this manner. Atopic dermatitis usually appears on the flexural surfaces of the body, and is less likely to have the raised borders seen in this picture. Contact dermatitis is usually vesicular.

303. The answer is a. (*McPhee, pp 121-123.*) Treatment for warts should be geared toward inducing "wart-free" intervals for as long as possible, and trying not to create scarring. No treatment can guarantee a remission or absolutely prevent reoccurrences. All the therapies listed in this question may be used for warts, but topical liquid nitrogen is the best choice in this case. Podophyllum resin should not be used during pregnancy. Imiquimod is often used for anogenital warts, but has not demonstrated benefit for common warts. Laser therapy is effective, but leaves open wounds that heal by secondary intention and should be reserved for warts resistant to other treatment modalities. Bleomycin injection has a high cure rate, but shouldn't be used on digital warts because of potential complications including terminal digital necrosis.

304. The answer is d. (*McPhee, pp 92-94.*) Atopic dermatitis or eczema may have a different appearance in different people. However, several characteristics do help to differentiate it from other causes of rash. The rash may look like rough, red plaques with some flaking that can affect the face, neck, upper trunk, and behind the knees. The flexural surfaces are often involved. Pruritus may be severe. Virtually all patients will have evidence of the disease before the age of 5 years, so a new diagnosis of atopic dermatitis in an adult should be made cautiously, and only after consultation.

305. The answer is c. (*South-Paul, pp 146-164.*) The lesion described is molluscum contagiosum. It can appear in individuals of all ages and all races, but is more commonly reported in white males. The lesion is due to an infection with a poxvirus transmitted through direct skin-to-skin contact. Lesions are common in children in a day-care or nursery school setting and are in that case not likely to be sexually transmitted. However, in adults and in the pubic region, they are sexually transmitted. Although the lesions can be similar to those seen with basal cell cancers, the lack of telangiectasia is a diagnostic clue. The lesions can occur in immunocompetent persons, but in patients who are immunocompromised, they are generally more numerous and larger. Most lesions will resolve spontaneously within months of appearance, but they can be treated with cryotherapy, cautery, or curettage.

306. The answer is e. (*Mengel, pp 332-338.*) The symptoms in this case are consistent with viral conjunctivitis. The presence of a palpable preauricular lymph node is characteristic of viral conjunctivitis. Approximately 85% of viral conjunctivitis is because of adenovirus, which is highly contagious, and is self-limited. Only 15% of conjunctivitis is bacterial. Characteristics of bacterial conjunctivitis include purulent discharge, pain, photophobia, and a "gritty" sensation of the eye. Topical corticosteroids are contraindicated in conjunctivitis, as studies have documented increased duration of viral shedding, prolongation of the infectious period, and potential corneal ulcerations and perforations. Antiviral eye drops are indicated for herpetic eye infections, but without corneal dendrites with fluorescein staining, that diagnosis is unlikely. The treatment for nonherpetic viral conjunctivitis is supportive, using cold compresses and lubricating drops.

307. The answer is e. (*Rakel, pp 230-233.*) Symptoms of conjunctivitis include increased redness, irritation, tearing, discharge, photophobia, or itching. Pain is more suggestive of a more serious problem, possibly a corneal abrasion or other pathology.

308. The answer is e. *(Rakel, pp 230-233.)* Of the symptoms of conjunctivitis, itching is more specific for allergic conditions. The other things listed (except for use of oral contraceptives) are more general and not useful in differentiating allergic conjunctivitis from other causes. The use of oral contraceptives may, in some people, cause a dry eye, but is less likely to cause conjunctivitis.

309. The answer is c. *(Rakel, pp 230-233.)* Adenovirus is the most common virus causing conjunctivitis. It can be transmitted through ocular and respiratory secretions, and less commonly from fomites on towels or equipment. It has an 8-day incubation period, and a 10- to 12-day viral shedding period. Supportive treatment is indicated.

310. The answer is d. *(Rakel, pp 230-233.)* Bacterial conjunctivitis is most commonly caused by *Streptococcus* and *Staphylococcus.* However, gram-negative organisms should be strongly suspected in contact lens wearers. Therefore, gentamicin is the medication of choice. If gram-negative organisms are not suspected, fluoroquinolones or polymyxin-trimethoprim can be used.

311. The answer is c. *(Mengel, pp 332-338. Rakel, pp 230-233.)* Gonococcal conjunctivitis is considered an ophthalmologic emergency because of this organism's propensity to cause corneal perforation. The patient will have a red, irritated eye with copious purulent discharge. After cleaning the eye, it reforms almost immediately. Initial therapy would include IV ceftriaxone along with topical fluoroquinolone or tobramycin therapy. One should also consider concurrent treatment for chlamydial conjunctivitis.

312. The answer is a. *(Rakel, pp 230-233.)* Scleritis is a unilateral diffuse injection of the deeper scleral vessels. Symptoms include decreased vision, deep "boring" eye pain and a surrounding headache. It is usually associated with systemic autoimmune diseases like rheumatoid arthritis or Wegener granulomatosis. Episcleritis is associated with mild irritation, and is not as intense as the syndrome described above. A corneal abrasion is associated with decreased vision, intense pain, and tearing, but is associated with trauma. Acute glaucoma is associated with pain, decreased vision, and redness, but the affected pupil is usually dilated. Iritis also has similar symptoms, but the pupil is small.

313. The answer is e. *(Rakel, pp 255-258.)* Despite the fact that rhinosinusitis is the most commonly reported chronic condition on health surveys, and despite the fact that it accounts for approximately 12% of all antibiotics prescribed in the United States, there is no specific sign or symptom that defines sinusitis. The most common symptoms are congestion, facial pressure, nasal discharge, dental pain, loss of smell, and headache. Persistence of symptoms beyond the usual 7- to 10-day course of a viral upper respiratory infection most commonly defines clinical rhinosinusitis.

314. The answer is a. *(Rakel, pp 255-258.)* While all of the conditions listed predispose to bacterial infections of the sinus cavities, allergic rhinitis is the most common one listed. It is present in at least 60% of people with recurrent sinusitis.

315. The answer is d. *(Rakel, pp 255-258.)* *Streptococcus pneumoniae* and nontypable *H influenzae* are the most commonly cultured organisms in radiographically documented acute sinusitis. *Moraxella catarrhalis* is cultured from approximately 20% of pediatric cases, but is more uncommon in adults. *Staphylococcus aureus* can be cultured from approximately 30% of healthy noses, but is uncommonly cultured in specimens obtained from acute sinusitis. Chronic sinusitis is more commonly polymicrobial.

316. The answer is d. *(Rakel, pp 255-258.)* Chronic sinusitis is classically defined as symptoms that persist beyond 3 months. However, the more common history is that of symptoms that improve with therapy then reoccur. In general, empirical therapy of adult chronic sinusitis should begin with fluoroquinolones or amoxicillin/clavulanate for 2 to 3 weeks. High-dose amoxicillin or a cephalosporin may also be considered, but for 14 to 21 days.

317. The answer is e. *(Rakel, pp 255-258.)* Decongestants such as phenylpropanolamine and pseudoephedrine have not been shown to change the course of clinical respiratory tract disease. α-Agonists have not been shown to shorten the course of sinusitis, and can lead to symptomatic rebound congestion after just 1 week of use. Echinacea has not been shown to prevent or to speed resolution of sinusitis. Topical nasal steroids are the most potent treatment for nasal congestion and have been shown to potentiate the treatment benefits of antibiotics in chronic sinusitis.

318. The answer is a. *(Rakel, pp 1218-1222.)* The injury described is called a "burner" or "stinger." They are very common in contact sports, and usually are sustained by a lateral flexion force distracting the head and shoulder away from the affected side, compression injury with the head and neck flexed toward the affected side, or a direct blow to the supraclavicular region. If symptoms resolve, and neck palpation and range of motion, shoulder and upper extremity neurological examination are all normal, patients can return to play. If both sides are involved, radiographs should be obtained to rule out cervical spine injury. An electromyography (EMG) can be obtained, but may take up to 3 weeks after the injury to become abnormal. Physical therapy may be useful for residual symptoms.

319. The answer is e. *(Rakel, pp 1218-1222.)* The injury described above is a type IV acromioclavicular separation. This is defined by more than a 50% separation of the joint with a posterior displacement of the clavicle. Treatment should be surgical. With less severe separations, treatment can be conservative—with sling immobilization, early range of motion exercises—and return to play when the pain subsides.

320. The answer is d. *(Rakel, pp 1218-1222.)* The patient described has patellofemoral syndrome, the most common overuse injury seen in the athlete under 40 years of age. While the mechanism is poorly understood, it is felt to be because of biomechanics, with the patella tracking laterally to the more developed vastus lateralis muscle. Patients complain of knee pain with use, but also note pain when the knee is held in flexion for long periods of time (the "movie theatre sign"). Treatment should be directed at stretching the hamstrings and building the vastus medialis muscle to improve biomechanics.

321. The answer is b. *(Rakel, pp 1218-1222.)* The twisting injury, feeling of a "pop," and immediate effusion while still being able to bear weight are consistent with an ACL tear. The sense of instability also helps lead toward that diagnosis. Patellofemoral pain would generally not occur acutely or after an injury. The mechanism of a posterior cruciate ligament injury is through direct force to the knee. Meniscal injuries also cause knee pain, but are more likely to cause locking, catching, or giving way. Collateral ligament tears would likely lead to more instability than that described in the question.

322. The answer is d. *(Rakel, pp 1218-1222.)* The test described is the McMurray test, and is positive when the maneuver elicits a catch or click with pain at the joint line, indicating a meniscal tear.

323. The answer is a. *(Rakel, pp 1218-1222.)* The Ottawa ankle rules are a useful guide to use to determine if radiographs are indicated after an ankle sprain. Films should be obtained if

- The patient is unable to walk four steps immediately after the injury and in the office.
- There is tenderness over the distal 6 cm of the tibia or fibula, including the malleoli.
- There is midfoot or navicular tenderness.
- There is tenderness over the proximal fifth metatarsal.

Rest, ice, compression, and elevation are mainstays of therapy, but the x-ray is imperative for this case. Early mobilization is recommended, unless there is a fracture present. NSAIDs should be reserved for 48 hours after an injury because it may exacerbate bleeding and swelling acutely. Physical therapy may help expedite return to activity in the long run, but only after fracture has been ruled out.

324. The answer is c. *(Mengel, pp 359-364.)* Studies have shown that a limited evaluation including a hematocrit, serum creatine kinase, glucose, ECG, carotid massage, orthostatic blood pressure, and evaluation of pulses yields a diagnosis of syncope in the majority of cases. Additional testing including a Holter monitor, echocardiogram, ambulatory loop ECG, and tilt table testing yields a diagnosis in an additional 5% of patients. All patients with syncope should have an ECG, even though the diagnostic yield is low. It is relatively easy, risk-free, and can help rule out the most concerning cardiac causes. A CBC (including WBC count and platelets) is probably not needed unless an infectious etiology is suspected, and a TSH assessment is also not necessary unless thyroid disease is suspected.

325. The answer is a. *(Mengel, pp 359-364.)* In syncopal patients who present with a heart murmur, echocardiography should be obtained. It will help rule out valvular heart disease, but will also identify hypertrophic cardiomyopathy (the likely cause in this question). Holter monitoring and long-term ambulatory loop ECG testing will help identify arrhythmias, stress testing will help identify ischemia and/or exercise-induced arrhythmias, and tilt table tests are indicated in patients with unexplained recurrent syncope in whom cardiac causes are ruled out.

326. The answer is d. *(Mengel, pp 359-364.)* The patient in this scenario had exertional dyspnea and diaphoresis. As a diabetic, she is at high risk for silent ischemia, often signaled by anginal equivalents such as dyspnea and diaphoresis. A hypoglycemic event could have also caused diaphoresis and syncope, but serum glucose testing 1 day later would not help identify that as a cause. In addition, glycosolated hemoglobin would not be helpful in determining the cause of the event. An echocardiogram would not be helpful without physical examination findings consistent with cardiomyopathy or valvular disease, and a Holter monitor would be less helpful without evidence of palpitations or ECG abnormalities.

327. The answer is e. *(Mengel, pp 359-364.)* Tilt table testing is recommended in patients with unexplained recurrent syncope in whom cardiac causes including arrhythmias have been ruled-out. An abnormal result suggests vasovagal syncope. Psychiatric evaluation should be considered if the tilt table is normal, especially if associated with other psychiatric symptoms (anxiety, depression, fear, or dread). Carotid Dopplers and MRI of the brain should be reserved for people with bruits or focal neurological signs. Stress testing is indicated if there is high risk for, or symptoms of ischemic disease.

328. The answer is b. *(McPhee, pp 637-639.)* The classic presentation of vaginal candidiasis is vaginal itch with white "cheesy" exudate. White plaques usually adhere to the vaginal wall. The KOH preparation shows multiple hyphae. Treatment consists of topical azole applications or an oral one-time dose of fluconazole. To date, no data prove oral medications to be superior to topical medications.

329. The answer is c. *(South-Paul, pp 146-164.)* Recurrent yeast infections have been erroneously ascribed to many causes. They probably do *not* occur more frequently in diabetic women, but may be more difficult to eradicate in this population. Similarly, women with HIV may manifest or present with diffuse candidiasis that is difficult to eradicate, but not with recurrent infections. There is no convincing evidence that birth control pills cause infections. High-calorie diets and crude fiber have been associated with susceptibility to infection. Although not a true sexually transmitted disease, when a patient has frequent relapses of vaginal candidiasis, treatment of the partner may be considered, especially if he has balanitis.

330. The answer is c. *(McPhee, pp 637-639.)* The history and physical described are classic for trichomonas vaginalis. The classic "strawberry cervix" is a strong diagnostic clue. Trichomonads are seen on high power in the saline preparation, and appear as triangular cells with long tails, slightly larger than WBC. "Studded" epithelial cells (clue cells) are more consistent with bacterial vaginosis, "moth-eaten" cells (pseudo-clue cells) are seen in an acid-base disturbance of the vagina. Numerous WBC are more consistent with an upper genital infection, and hyphae are consistent with vaginal candidiasis.

331. The answer is a. (*McPhee, pp 637-639.*) The condition described is bacterial vaginosis. Clue cells, epithelial cells studded with bacteria, are diagnostically helpful. The treatment of choice is topical or oral metronidazole, with oral or topical clindamycin being an acceptable alternative. Doxycycline is used to treat *Chlamydia*. Clotrimazole is used to treat fungal infections. Imiquimod is an immunomodulating agent approved to treat HPV infection, and acyclovir treats herpetic infections.

332. The answer is a. (*Mengel, pp 396-400.*) Acute viral respiratory tract infections cause up to 50% of wheezing episodes in children less than 2 years of age. Risk factors include fall or winter season, history of atopy, day-care attendance, and passive smoke exposure. Pneumonia causes 33% to 50% of wheezing episodes in children, and most are also caused by viruses as well. Bronchiolitis accounts for less than 5% of all episodes of wheezing, but is important, especially in preterm infants. Aspiration is uncommon, and is less likely in the setting of viral infection symptoms. Asthma is common in children, but is not diagnosed after one episode of wheezing.

333. The answer is d. (*Mengel, pp 396-400.*) Wheezing is commonly heard in patients with CHF. Risk factors include hypertension, glucose intolerance, and smoking. Treatment should begin with diuresis. Antibiotics would be prescribed for an infection, epinephrine for a suspected allergic reaction, steroids for an asthma exacerbation, and anticoagulation if a PE is suspected.

334. The answer is c. (*Mengel, pp 396-400.*) When a patient presents with acute shortness of breath and an increased respiratory rate, PE must be ruled out. The patient in this case is taking oral contraceptives, increasing her risk for PE. After appropriate workup, anticoagulation should be initiated. An allergic reaction, asthma or bronchitis would likely cause an abnormal lung examination.

335. The answer is b. (*Mengel, pp 396-400.*) Patients with a first episode of wheezing require a chest x-ray. Peak flow testing may be helpful in monitoring control of asthma, but are not useful in evaluating a first episode.

Pulmonary function testing and a CBC may be needed, but a chest x-ray is an absolute necessity.

336. The answer is e. *(Mengel, pp 396-400.)* The patient described likely has GERD, a common cause of wheezing in the pediatric population. The gold standard test is a 24-hour pH probe. Endoscopy is invasive, requires sedation, and is usually reserved for patients unresponsive to medical management. A chest x-ray is unlikely to reveal the cause in this case, and a barium swallow is indicated if the physician is concerned about structural defects. Pulmonary function testing is difficult in this age group.

337. The answer is b. *(Mengel, pp 396-400.)* In patients with known asthma, chest x-rays are not required to evaluate each episode. A chest x-ray is indicated if the patient has fever, rhonchi, or sputum to rule out pneumonia. Peak flows do not confirm the diagnosis of asthma, but are useful to monitor the status of known lung disease. Pulmonary function tests may be needed, but are usually done in a pulmonary laboratory. A CBC may indicate infection, but would be less useful in this setting. Nasopharyngeal washes may be helpful in the pediatric population, but are not as helpful for adults.

Chronic Conditions

Questions

338. A 42-year-old male is seeing you to discuss sexual concerns. He complains of being unable to achieve an erection, despite having strong interest in sexual activity. Which of the following is true?

a. This is most often because of an unrecognized mood disorder
b. This is most often because of a lack of attraction for his partner
c. This is most often because of stressors in the home and interpersonal conflict
d. This is most often because of a vascular problem
e. This is most often because of alcohol abuse

339. A 36-year-old man sees you to discuss a lack of sexual interest. He is not having sexual fantasies and is unmotivated to begin sexual activity. He does not report depressive symptoms and has no other physical complaints. His physical examination is normal. Which of the following laboratory tests is most appropriate?

a. Total testosterone
b. Free testosterone
c. Thyroid-stimulating hormone (TSH)
d. Prolactin
e. Prostate specific antigen (PSA)

340. You are caring for a 45-year-old man with hypertension, gastroesophageal reflux, and depression. His medication list includes hydrochlorothiazide, verapamil, lisinopril, omeprazole, fluoxetine, and trazodone. He is complaining of difficulty with ejaculation. Which of the following medications is the most likely cause of this problem?

a. Hydrochlorothiazide
b. Verapamil
c. Lisinopril
d. Omeprazole
e. Fluoxetine

341. You have diagnosed a 30-year-old woman with depression. She is concerned that medical treatment may cause sexual dysfunction. In order to avoid sexual side-effects, which antidepressant would be the best choice?

a. Amitriptyline
b. Paroxetine
c. Citalopram
d. Sertraline
e. Bupropion

342. A 23-year-old man comes to your office to discuss premature ejaculation. He has had this condition since beginning sexual activity at 17 years of age. He has tried behavioral methods, but these have not been successful. Which of the following medications is most likely to help this condition?

a. Alprostadil
b. Fluoxetine
c. Bupropion
d. Silendafil
e. Atenolol

343. You are considering androgen replacement in a 50-year-old man with decreased sexual desire. Which of the following preparations would result in the most consistent levels and the fewest side-effects?

a. Oral testosterone replacement
b. Intramuscular testosterone injection
c. Topical testosterone patches
d. Topical testosterone gel
e. Sublingual testosterone

344. You are seeing a 61-year-old patient and are concerned about substance abuse. He is single, employed as a lawyer in an extremely stressful job. Which of the following characteristics are most likely to increase his risk for a substance use disorder?

a. His age
b. His marital status
c. His job as a lawyer
d. His job stress level
e. His level of education

✓ **345.** You are evaluating a 28-year-old man who is concerned about depression. He reports increased irritability, depressed mood, decreased enjoyment from usual activities, and sleep and appetite disturbances for 6 weeks. He reports a history of alcohol use, and currently has 6 beers a day on the weekdays, with up to 12 on the weekends. Which of the following is the most appropriate next step in treating his depression?

a. Treat with a selective serotonin reuptake inhibitor (SSRI)
b. Treat with bupropion
c. Recommend detoxification and abstinence
d. Recommend detoxification and abstinence and start an SSRI
e. Recommend detoxification and abstinence and start bupropion

346. You suspect that a 50-year-old female patient is abusing alcohol. Which of the following is the most sensitive laboratory test to confirm this?

a. Mean corpuscular volume (MCV)
b. Alanine aminotransferase (ALT)
c. Aspartate aminotransferase (AST)
d. γ-Glutamyl transferase (GGT)
e. Lactate dehydrogenase (LDH)

347. You suspect that a 56-year-old male patient is abusing alcohol. Which of the following is the most specific laboratory test to confirm this?

a. MCV
b. ALT
c. AST
d. GGT
e. LDH

348. An alcoholic patient of yours is interested in pharmacologic therapy to help him with his sobriety. His counselor recommended he try naltrexone, and he asks you how that medication works in alcoholism. Which of the following is the best answer for your patient?

a. If the person taking naltrexone ingests alcohol, it causes an adverse reaction.
b. Naltrexone reduces the reinforcing effects of alcohol.
c. Naltrexone blocks the effects of alcohol by binding to alcohol-receptor sites on cells.
d. Naltrexone saturates the alcohol-receptor sites on cells by acting as an alcohol agonist.
e. Naltrexone changes the binding sites on alcohol, making it unable to bind to cells.

349. An alcoholic patient of yours is interested in pharmacologic therapy to help him in his sobriety. His counselor recommended he try disulfiram, and he asks you how that medication works in alcoholism. Which of the following is the best answer for your patient?

a. If the person taking disulfiram ingests alcohol, it causes an adverse reaction.
b. Disulfiram reduces the reinforcing effects of alcohol.
c. Disulfiram blocks the effects of alcohol by binding to alcohol receptor sites on cells.
d. Disulfiram saturates the alcohol receptor sites on cells by acting as an alcohol agonist.
e. Disulfiram changes the binding sites on alcohol, making it unable to bind to cells.

350. Your patient asks you about pharmacotherapy to help him to prevent relapse of alcohol abuse. Which of the following medications is most effective for this purpose?

a. Disulfiram
b. Naltrexone
c. Serotonergic drugs
d. Acamprosate
e. Tricyclics

√**351.** A 33-year-old male patient is seeing you for advice on how to quit smoking. He has tried many times in the past and has been unsuccessful. Which of the following symptoms characterizes the nicotine-withdrawal syndrome?

a. Hypersomnolence
b. Depressed mood
c. Psychomotor retardation
d. Lethargy
e. Amotivational syndrome

352. You are caring for a patient who would like to quit smoking. She failed nicotine patches. Which of the following is an appropriate next step?

a. Add nicotine gum to the patch
b. Use clonidine
c. Use a tricyclic antidepressant
d. Use a SSRI
e. Use a selective serotonin and norepinephrine reuptake inhibitor

353. Your patient is thinking of using varenicline (Chantix) to help with smoking cessation. Which of the following is true of this medication?

a. Varenicline has many drug interactions.
b. The dose of this medication would need to be changed in patients with liver disease.
c. Common side effects include abnormal dreams.
d. This medication is contraindicated in patients with a seizure disorder.
e. Patients cannot smoke while taking varenicline.

354. You are currently evaluating a patient for unstable angina. He takes phenytoin for a seizure disorder, has high cholesterol and is a current smoker. Which of the following would be the best pharmacotherapeutic option to help with his smoking cessation plan?

a. Behavioral intervention
b. Nicotine replacement
c. Bupropion
d. Varenicline
e. Clonidine

355. In a preemployment screen, one of your patients tested positive for cocaine use. He presents to you and would like to discontinue his use, but reports having significant problems with the withdrawal symptoms. Which of the following symptoms is expected from cocaine-withdrawal?

a. Tachycardia
b. Hypertension
c. Depression
d. Paranoia
e. Insomnia

356. You are caring for a 35-year-old woman in the hospital, admitted for cellulitis. She also has a long history of migraine headaches. On day 2 of her hospitalization, she becomes diaphoretic, restless, and irritable. Within hours, she is complaining of severe pain, abdominal cramps, and diarrhea. Which of the following would most likely be present in her urine toxicology screen?

a. Cocaine
b. Marijuana
c. Opiates
d. 3,4-Methylenedioxymethampheatmine (MDMA or ecstasy)
e. Benzodiazepines

357. A 64-year-old woman comes to see you as a new patient. She is interested in finding the cause of her hand deformities. Upon inspection, you see the joints in her hands are nodular and enlarged as in the picture below:

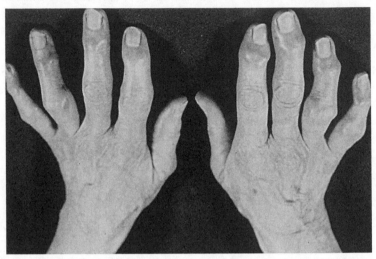

(Reproduced, with permission, from South-Paul J. Current Diagnosis and Treatment in Family Medicine, *1st ed. New York: McGraw-Hill, 2004:266.)*

Which of the following laboratory findings is likely in her case?

a. Her laboratory evaluation will likely be normal
b. Her serum uric acid level will likely be elevated
c. Her sedimentation rate will likely be elevated
d. Her C-reactive protein level will likely be elevated
e. Her rheumatoid factor will likely be elevated

358. You are evaluating a 62-year-old man who is complaining of joint pain. His pain involves his left knee, right ankle, and both hands. He reports that his symptoms have been present for years, but are worsening. He has more pain with activity. On examination, you note some swelling in the joints with mild tenderness and crepitus. Which of the following is the most likely cause of his symptoms?

a. Rheumatoid arthritis
b. Osteoarthritis
c. Gout
d. Tendonitis
e. Fibromyalgia

√**359.** A 43-year-old obese patient comes to your office with a painful, inflamed, swollen elbow. He reports that the pain began suddenly last evening, without a known precipitant or trauma. The pain is exquisite, and does not allow him to move his elbow at all—in fact, even the pressure of his bed sheet on his elbow was painful. On examination, he has an elbow effusion with warmth, erythema, and intense pain with movement. Which of the following is most likely the cause?

a. Rheumatoid arthritis
b. Osteoarthritis
c. Gout
d. Stress fracture
e. Cellulitis

√**360.** You are caring for a 31-year-old woman who complains of joint pain. She notes that her hands seem to be stiff in the morning, and that she seems to improve with time, movement, and heat. She reports more fatigue than usual as well. On examination, her wrists are swollen bilaterally, as are several of her metacarpal-phalangeal joints on each hand. Which of the following is her most likely diagnosis?

a. Rheumatoid arthritis
b. Osteoarthritis
c. Gout
d. Tendonitis
e. Fibromyalgia

361. A 70-year-old man with diabetes and long-term osteoarthritis in his knees is presenting for follow-up. He reports that his pain has become much more severe, and says he is having difficulty with ambulation and is becoming fairly inactive. In the past, he tried ibuprofen and naproxen, but those offered limited improvement and he developed secondary ulcers. He says that taking acetaminophen is like "taking a sugar pill"— it offers no help. He had some relief from steroid injections 3 months ago, and again 1 month ago, but they were short-lived. A recent x-ray is shown below:

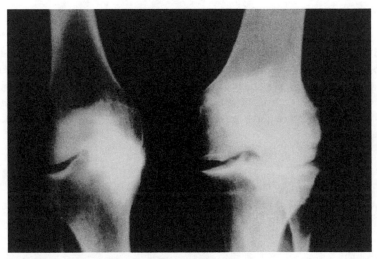

(Reproduced, with permission, from South-Paul J. Current Diagnosis and Treatment in Family Medicine, *1st ed. New York: McGraw-Hill, 2004:267.)*

Which of the following is the next most appropriate step in the treatment of his condition?

a. Use oral steroids
b. Try another steroid injection
c. Inject the knee joint with ketorolac (Toradol)
d. Inject hyaluronic acid into his knee joints
e. Refer for knee replacements

362. You are caring for a 50-year-old man who reports frequent episodes of gout. He drinks two to three glasses of wine with dinner each night. Which of the following is true regarding the relationship between alcohol and gout?

a. Alcohol causes the release of uric acid from the liver.
b. Alcohol itself increases crystal formation in the joint.
c. Alcohol alters renal excretion of uric acid.
d. Alcohol contains relatively large quantities of uric acid.
e. Alcohol contains sulfites that metabolize into uric acid after absorption in the gut.

363. A 66-year-old diabetic man comes to your office with acute monoarticular arthritis. You suspect gout. Which of the following tests is the most helpful in establishing the diagnosis?

a. Sedimentation rate
b. C-reactive protein
c. Serum uric acid levels
d. Evaluation of joint aspirate
e. Twenty-four-hour urine collection to measure uric acid excretion

364. You are evaluating a patient with knee swelling and pain. You perform an arthrocentesis to help determine the diagnosis. The fluid analysis reveals rhomboid-shaped positively birefringent crystals. Which of the following is the most likely diagnosis?

a. Gout
b. Pseudogout
c. Infectious arthritis
d. Osteoarthritis
e. Rheumatoid arthritis

365. You are evaluating a patient with a painful, swollen knee. You perform arthrocentesis to find cloudy fluid. Analysis reveals a white blood cell (WBC) count of 50,000/mm^3 with more than 90% identified as polymorphonuclear (PMN) leukocytes. The glucose level in the joint fluid is decreased. Which of the following is the most likely diagnosis?

a. Gout
b. Pseudogout
c. Infectious arthritis
d. Osteoarthritis
e. Rheumatoid arthritis

√ **366.** You are evaluating a patient with a painful, swollen knee. Joint aspirate reveals clear fluid with a WBC count of 5000/mm³, 20% of which are PMN leukocytes. Which of the following is the most likely diagnosis?

a. Gout
b. Pseudogout
c. Infectious arthritis
d. Osteoarthritis
e. Rheumatoid arthritis

√ **367.** The joint aspirate from the inflamed first metatarsal-phalangeal joint of a 35-year-old woman reveals needle-shaped negatively birefringent crystals. The patient is intolerant to nonsteroidals. Which of the following is the most appropriate initial treatment?

a. Colchicine
b. Corticosteroids
c. Opiates
d. Allopurinol
e. Probenecid

368. You are following a 52-year-old woman with stiff, swollen hands. Her left hand is shown below:

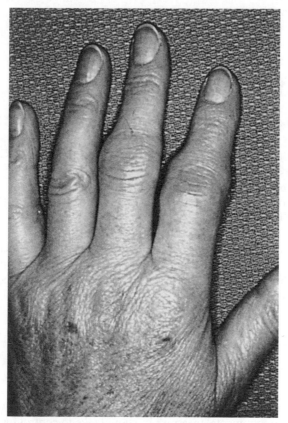

(Reproduced, with permission, from South-Paul J. Current Diagnosis and Treatment in Family Medicine, *1st ed. New York: McGraw-Hill, 2004:276.)*

Her right hand is similar. She describes prolonged morning symptoms, and excessive fatigue. Based on this information, which of the following is the most likely diagnosis?

a. Osteoarthritis
b. Gout
c. Tophaceous gout
d. Rheumatoid arthritis
e. Systemic lupus erythematosis

369. You are caring for a 42-year-old woman who was diagnosed with rheumatoid arthritis (RA) 8 years ago. You are concerned about potential extra-articular manifestations of her disease. Which of the following signs or symptoms, if present, would signal extra-articular manifestations RA?

a. Cough
b. Congestive heart failure (CHF)
c. Gastrointestinal (GI) distress
d. Peripheral neuropathy
e. Renal failure

370. You have recently determined that a patient in your office has RA. Which of the following is the most appropriate next step?

a. Control symptoms with nonsteroidal anti-inflammatory drugs (NSAIDs)
b. Control symptoms with opiates
c. Use steroid treatment for flares, and NSAIDs for daily use
d. Use steroid injections to keep flares under control
e. Refer to rheumatology

371. You are seeing a patient in the office for the first time. She has had recent episodic shortness of breath and is concerned that she has developed asthma. Which of the following features, if present, is the strongest predisposing factor in the development of asthma?

a. Family history of asthma
b. History of atopy
c. A history of childhood pneumonia
d. Exposure to cigarette smoke
e. Exposure to environmental pollution

372. You have recently diagnosed a 24-year-old man with asthma. You are discussing environmental measures he should take to control his symptoms and avoid triggers. Which of the following is the most appropriate advice?

a. Keep humidity in the home relatively high, above 50%
b. Enclose his mattress and pillows with allergen impermeable covers
c. Launder bed linens with cold water
d. Install carpeting if possible
e. Use air filters to decrease the levels of dust mite allergens

373. You are seeing a 19-year-old college student complaining of recurrent and persistent cough. She has been treated for "bronchitis" several times, and you are concerned that her true diagnosis is asthma. Which of the following is most important in the diagnosis of asthma?

a. History
b. Allergy testing
c. Chest x-ray
d. Pulmonary function tests with and without bronchodilator therapy
e. Provocative testing with methocholine

✓**374.** You are caring for a 30-year-old woman who has had asthma since childhood. Currently, she reports symptoms three or four times a week, but never more than once a day. Sometimes her symptoms cause her to skip her usual exercise regimen. She wakes in the night approximately three or four times a month to use her inhaler and return to bed. Which of the following classifications best characterizes her asthma?

a. Mild intermittent
b. Moderate intermittent
c. Mild persistent
d. Moderate persistent
e. Severe persistent

Review
Asthma
Diagnoses!

375. You are caring for an 18-year-old man with asthma. He smokes, and reports needing to use his short-acting bronchodilator daily. He gets flares of asthma at least twice a week, and while some days are relatively symptom-free, some exacerbations may last several days. He wakes up at least once a week with symptoms. Which of the following classifications best characterizes his asthma?

a. Mild intermittent
b. Moderate intermittent
c. Mild persistent
d. Moderate persistent
e. Severe persistent

376. You are discussing asthma control with a 22-year-old patient. She monitors her therapy closely, and reports that her current peak flows are at about 80% of her best levels. Which of the following is the best approach to take at this point?

a. Commend the patient on her diligent monitoring and excellent control.
b. Reassure the patient that this is well within the normal range.
c. Review the patient's medications and technique and review environmental control.
d. Have the patient take additional medication, or add a medication to her regimen.
e. Consider hospitalization.

377. You are caring for a young woman who has had mild intermittent asthma for years. She uses a short-acting bronchodilator as needed, but in the past has only needed therapy once or twice a month. Over the past 2 months, she has noted that she is using her inhaler more. In fact, she uses it at least three times a week, and on occasion has had to wake up in the middle of the night to use her inhaler. Which of the following is the most appropriate treatment option at this point?

a. Change her short-acting β-agonist from albuterol (Proventil, Ventolin) to pirbuterol (Maxair)
b. Add a long-acting β-agonist
c. Add an inhaled corticosteroid
d. Add a leukotriene receptor antagonist
e. Add cromolyn (Intal)

378. You are caring for a man with asthma. He is currently taking an inhaled corticosteroid twice daily and using his short-acting β-agonist as needed. Over the past 3 months, he has required escalating doses of his inhaled corticosteroid, and now he is at the maximum dosage, still using his "rescue" inhaler more than he would like. Which of the following is the best medication to add to his regimen?

a. A burst and rapid taper of oral steroids
b. A long-acting β-agonist
c. Cromolyn (Intal)
d. Ipratropium (Atrovent)
e. Theophylline

✓ **379.** You are caring for a 19-year-old man who has been treated for mild intermittent asthma since childhood. He has been controlled using a short-acting bronchodilator as needed. Over the past month, he has been using his inhaler more than four times a week, and has had to wake up in the middle of the night to use his inhaler on three occasions. In the past, he was intolerant of the side-effects associated with an inhaled corticosteroid. Which of the following is the most appropriate treatment option?

a. Long-acting β-agonist
b. Leukotriene receptor antagonist
c. Cromolyn (Intal)
d. Theophylline
e. Oral corticosteroids

✓ **380.** A 22-year-old man is seeing you to discuss his low back pain. He is athletic and exercises regularly. He denies any inciting event, does not have pain with movement, and denies radiation of the pain. Given this information, which of the following is the most likely diagnosis?

a. Spondylolisthesis
b. Low back strain
c. Degenerative osteoarthritis
d. Lumbar disk herniation
e. Neoplasm

✓ **381.** You are seeing a 40-year-old woman who reports the gradual onset of low back pain over several months. The pain is associated with morning stiffness that improves throughout the day. On examination, there are no neurological deficits. Which of the following is the most likely cause?

a. Back strain
b. Inflammatory arthropathy
c. Disk herniation
d. Compression fracture
e. Neoplasm

382. You are evaluating a 41-year-old man with the acute onset of low back pain. It started 2 days ago while he was putting his child into his car seat. The pain radiates to his right leg. On examination, his range of motion is limited but his neurological examination is normal. When you lay him on his back and raise his fully extended leg about 30° by the heel, he reports pain below the knee. Which of the following is the most likely diagnosis?

a. Back strain
b. An inflammatory condition
c. Disk herniation
d. Compression fracture
e. Neoplasm

383. A 41-year-old sedentary man presented to you 6 weeks ago with the acute onset of low back pain radiating to the left leg. His neurological examination at the time was normal, but he did not respond to conservative therapy. X-rays are normal. Which of the following is the most appropriate next step?

a. Flexion and extension radiographs
b. Magnetic resonance imaging (MRI)
c. Electromyelography
d. Bone scan
e. A complete blood count (CBC) and erythrocyte sedimentation rate (ESR)

384. A 30-year-old woman was putting her groceries into her trunk and noted the sudden onset of low back pain. She has tried acetaminophen for 2 days without relief. On examination, her range of motion is limited, and she has tenderness to palpation of the lumbar paraspinal muscles. Which of the following treatment options is best?

a. NSAIDs and return to normal activity
b. Opiate analgesia and limited activities
c. Oral corticosteroids
d. Bed rest for 3 to 5 days
e. Spinal traction

385. You are evaluating a 31-year-old man complaining of left-sided neck and upper back pain. He reports worsening discomfort when he turns his head toward the left, with some paresthesias in his left upper extremity. On examination, when you rotate his head to the left and exert downward pressure on his head, it reproduces the pain and paresthesia. Which of the following is the most likely diagnosis?

a. Cervical strain
b. Cervical disk herniation
c. Torticollis
d. Spondylosis
e. Osteoarthritis

386. A 60-year-old woman was the restrained driver in a motor vehicle accident yesterday. Today, she presents to you for evaluation. She reports neck and upper back pain. On examination, she does not have bony tenderness, but cannot rotate her head 45° to the right or left. Which of the following is the most appropriate next step?

a. Reassurance and NSAIDs
b. Cervical spine x-rays
c. MRI
d. Bone scan
e. Dual energy x-ray absorptiometry (DEXA) scan

387. You are assessing a 59-year-old patient with an 80-pack-year history of smoking cigarettes. He stopped smoking 1 year ago. He reports a cough productive of white frothy sputum for the past 4 months. Reviewing his chart, you discover that he had a similar presentation last winter, with a cough that lasted more than 3 months. Given this information, which of the following is his most likely diagnosis?

a. Asthma
b. Chronic bronchitis
c. Bronchiectasis
d. Emphysema
e. Recurrent pneumonia

388. You have been treating a 33-year-old woman for asthma for the last 3 years. She began with mild symptoms, but has become progressively more short of breath over the last year. She reports weight loss and significant dyspnea on exertion. She has never smoked, but her husband smokes in the home. Her maternal aunt was a smoker, and died of emphysema in her early 50s. Her chest x-ray reveals flattened diaphragms, a long, narrow heart cardiac silhouette, and increased retrosternal airspace on the lateral projection. Given this clinical picture and x-ray, which of the following is the most likely consideration?

a. Human immunodeficiency virus (HIV) with chronic lung infection
b. CHF
c. Chronic bronchitis
d. Lung cancer due to passive exposure to cigarette smoking
e. α_1-Antitrypsin deficiency

389. You have diagnosed a 66-year-old female patient of yours with chronic obstructive pulmonary disease (COPD). Which of the following therapies has been shown to improve the natural history of COPD?

a. Smoking cessation
b. Bronchodilators
c. Inhaled steroids
d. Antibiotics
e. Supplemental oxygen

390. You are caring for a 68-year-old smoker who complains of increasing shortness of breath with exertion and at rest. You observe that he is somewhat "barrel-chested," he breathes with pursed lips, and leans forward resting on his elbows when sitting in your office. On examination, he has decreased breath sounds and distant heart sounds. You are concerned about COPD and order office spirometry. Which of the following measurements is most sensitive to diagnose COPD?

a. Total lung capacity (TLC)
b. Forced vital capacity (FVC)
c. Forced expiratory volume in 1 second (FEV_1)
d. Forced expiratory flow rate over the interval from 25% to 75% of the total FVC ($FEF_{25\%-75\%}$)
e. FEV_1:FVC ratio

391. You are obtaining a family history from a new patient, and trying to determine her risk for various health conditions. She reports that her grandmother died of renal failure, but is unsure why her grandmother had that problem. Which of the following is the most common cause of end-stage renal disease?

a. Hypertensive nephropathy
b. Diabetic nephropathy
c. Polycystic kidney disease
d. Glomerulonephritis
e. Contrast-induced nephropathy

392. You are seeing a 65-year-old woman with a history of diabetes and hypertension. She is overweight and does not exercise regularly. You are concerned that she may have renal failure, given her risk factors. Which of the following is the best test to detect the presence of renal insufficiency in this patient?

a. Her blood urea nitrogen (BUN) level
b. Her serum creatinine level
c. Her BUN to creatinine ratio
d. Her calculated or estimated glomerular filtration rate (GFR)
e. Her urine microalbumin level

393. You are following a 54-year-old woman with diabetes. She has been very "brittle" and difficult to control. You are monitoring her urine microalbumin level and want to be alert to other changes that would suggest chronic renal insufficiency. If the patient were to develop chronic renal failure, which laboratory abnormality would you most likely see first?

a. Hyperkalemia
b. Hyponatremia
c. Hyperphosphatemia
d. Fall in plasma bicarbonate level
e. Anemia

394. You are following a 56-year-old Caucasian patient who has been diagnosed with hypertension and diabetes for 4 years. He does fairly well with diet and exercise, and has remained compliant with his medications. Laboratory evaluation demonstrates a normal serum creatinine, no microalbuminuria, but a GFR of 70 mL/min. According to the National Kidney Foundation staging guidelines, what stage of renal failure does this represent?

a. Stage 0 renal failure
b. Stage 1 renal failure
c. Stage 2 renal failure
d. Stage 3 renal failure
e. Stage 4 renal failure

395. You are seeing a 43-year-old hypertensive patient in your office. He is well-controlled with hydrochlorothiazide, and is seeing you for a routine evaluation. His blood pressure at the visit is 118/76 mm Hg. Laboratory evaluation reveals a normal creatinine and a GFR greater than 90 mL/min, but he does have microalbuminuria. Which of the following interventions is indicated in this patient?

a. Commend him on his excellent control and make no changes
b. Work to achieve better blood pressure control through diet and exercise
c. Increase his hydrochlorothiazide dose
d. Add an angiotensin-converting enzyme (ACE) inhibitor
e. Check a glycosolated hemoglobin level

396. You are following a 54-year-old patient with hypertension and diabetes in your office. Despite good blood pressure and glycemic control, his GFR has started to decrease. GFR measurement was 74 mL/min 3 months ago. At this visit, GFR is 55 mL/min. Creatinine is within normal limits, and his serum potassium is 5.2 mmol/L (normal is up to 5.1 mmol/L). The patient denies any changes in urination or other problems. Which of the following is most appropriate at this stage?

a. See the patient more frequently, at least monthly
b. Increase his ACE inhibitor
c. Add diuretic therapy
d. Refer to a nephrologist
e. Refer to a transplant surgeon

✓**397.** You are following a patient who is known to have primary biliary cirrhosis. You are following his liver function tests as indicators of disease severity and progression. Which of the following tests, if rising, would be most suggestive of a poor prognosis?

a. AST
b. ALT
c. GGT
d. Alkaline phosphatase
e. Bilirubin

✓ **398.** You are seeing a new patient in the office. His medical history is significant for cirrhosis. On examination, he has a significant fluid bulge at his flanks and a positive fluid wave. His laboratory tests reveal hyponatremia. Which of the following is the most likely cause of hyponatremia in this patient?

a. High levels of antidiuretic hormone secretion
b. Hepatic synthetic protein dysfunction causes osmotic losses of sodium
c. Shunting of blood away from the kidney to the liver
d. First-pass excretion of sodium
e. Osmotic sodium shifts from the blood to the ascitic fluid

399. You are seeing a new patient. He is 46 years old and has a significant history of alcohol use. He has several physical examination findings that are consistent with a potential diagnosis of cirrhosis. Which of the following is the best diagnostic test to confirm cirrhosis?

a. Computed tomography (CT) scan of the abdomen
b. Ultrasound of the abdomen
c. MRI of the abdomen
d. Radionuclide testing
e. Liver biopsy

400. You are evaluating a 48-year-old man with liver disease. His laboratory evaluation is as follows:

AST:	298 U/L (H)
ALT:	144 U/L (H)
Alk Phos:	140 U/L (H)
Bilirubin:	2.3 mg/dL (H)
GGT:	220 U/L (H)

Which of the following is the most likely cause of his liver disease?

a. Autoimmune hepatitis
b. Hepatitis B
c. Hepatitis C
d. Hematochromatosis
e. Alcoholic hepatitis

401. You are evaluating a 45-year-old man with liver disease. His laboratory evaluation reveals the following:

AST:	52 U/L (H)
ALT:	56 U/L (H)
Alkaline phosphatase:	132 U/L (H)
GGT:	188 U/L (H)
Albumin:	2.9 g/dL (L)
Bilirubin:	3.5 mg/dL (H)
Prothrombin time:	14.9 seconds (H)

Which of his lab results suggests that his liver disease is chronic?

a. AST
b. ALT
c. GGT
d. Alkaline phosphatase
e. Albumin

402. You care for a patient who contracted hepatitis C after a blood transfusion many years ago. Her liver disease has progressed, and she now has end-stage disease. Which of the following will be the most likely cause of death in this patient?

a. Liver failure
b. Hepatocellular carcinoma
c. Bleeding varices
d. Encephalopathy
e. Renal failure

403. You are taking care of a 47-year-old woman with cirrhosis. She asks you about transplantation as a definitive treatment option. Which of the following is an absolute contraindication to transplantation?

a. Active alcoholism
b. Portal vein thrombosis
c. Hepatitis B surface antigen positivity
d. HIV positivity
e. Extensive previous abdominal surgery

404. You are caring for a patient, who continues to smoke despite having asthma. She also has poorly controlled diabetes and hypertension with left ventricular hypertrophy. She presents to your office with shortness of breath. On physical examination, she appears to be in mild respiratory distress, and has 2+ pitting edema bilaterally. She has inspiratory and expiratory wheezes bilaterally, with dullness to percussion at the bases of her lungs. You order a stat b-type natriuretic peptide (BNP) and it comes back elevated at 498 pg/mL (normal is less than 100 pg/mL). Which of the following is the most likely diagnosis?

a. Asthma exacerbation
b. Pneumonia
c. CHF
d. Pulmonary embolus
e. Aspiration

405. You have diagnosed a 66-year-old woman with heart failure. She has a history of hypertension, but has never had heart failure before. Which of the following tests is routinely indicated in the initial evaluation of a person with a new diagnosis of heart failure?

a. Echocardiogram
b. Holter monitor
c. Left heart catheterization
d. Treadmill stress test
e. Pharmacologic stress test

406. You are seeing a patient she was discharged from the hospital. She initially presented to the emergency room with dyspnea and was found to be in CHF. They admitted her for diuresis and initiation of appropriate first-line therapy. Since being released, she reports that she is comfortable at rest, but that ordinary activity results in mild dyspnea. According to the NYHA functional classification, which class of heart failure best describes this patient?

a. Class I
b. Class II
c. Class III
d. Class IV
e. Class V

407. A 62-year-old woman comes to your office complaining of dyspnea. She has a history of COPD, hypertension, and diabetes. She also smokes and drinks heavily. Her evaluation reveals that she is in heart failure. Which of the following interventions will lead to functional improvement in this patient?

a. Optimizing the treatment of her COPD
b. Optimizing the treatment of her hypertension
c. Optimizing her glycemic control
d. Discontinuing cigarette smoking
e. Discontinuing alcohol use

408. You have diagnosed a 49-year-old man with CHF because of left ventricular systolic dysfunction. In addition to acute diuresis, which of the following is the best first-line agent to use for treatment, in the absence of contraindications?

a. ACE inhibitors
b. β-Blockers
c. Calcium channel blockers
d. Nitrates
e. Hydralazine

409. You have been treating a 68-year-old man suffering from chronic CHF with furosemide (Lasix), a β-blocker, and an ACE inhibitor. Despite this therapy, he continues with refractory edema. In his baseline state, he is comfortable at rest, but experiences some symptoms of heart failure with ordinary activity. Which of the following would be the best diuretic to add?

a. Hydrochlorothiazide
b. Triamterene
c. Hydrochlorothiazide and triamterene combined (Dyazide, Maxzide)
d. Metolazone (Zaroxolyn)
e. Spironolactone (Aldactone)

410. Which of the following statements is true regarding the use of angiotensin II receptor blockers (ARBs) in CHF?

a. ARBs and ACE inhibitors have the same effects on the neurohormonal mechanisms involved in heart failure.
b. Adding an ARB to an ACE inhibitor reduces mortality in patients with CHF.
c. Adding an ARB to an ACE inhibitor can reduce hospitalizations in patients with CHF.
d. Using an ARB instead of an ACE inhibitor increases mortality in CHF.
e. Using an ARB instead of an ACE inhibitor increases hospitalizations in patients with CHF.

411. You are treating a patient for heart failure because of systolic dysfunction with daily diuretics and an ACE inhibitor. He is continuing to have symptoms with activity, but they do not seem to be related to volume overload. Adding which of the following medications has been shown to reduce symptoms and improve mortality?

a. Metolazone (Zaroxolyn)
b. Spironolactone (Aldactone)
c. Metoprolol (Toprol XL)
d. Nifedipine (Procardia)
e. Digoxin (Lanoxin)

412. You take care of a 56-year-old woman whose 75-year-old mother just began living with her. The mother has been given a presumptive diagnosis of Alzheimer disease. The daughter is trying to learn all she can about the illness and asks you what causes it. Which of the following is believed to be the critical pathologic problem involved in Alzheimer disease?

a.   Brain atrophy
b.   Destruction of neurons
c.   Edema of neurons
d.   Shrinkage of large cortical neurons
e.   Loss of synapses

413. Which of the following is the most consistent neurochemical change associated with Alzheimer disease?

a.   Deficiency in glutamate
b.   Decline in cholinergic activity
c.   Decreased norepinephrine levels
d.   Increased somatostatin levels
e.   Increased corticotropin-releasing factor activity

414. You are concerned that one of your 65-year-old patients is developing dementia. Which of the following, if present, would lead you to suspect dementia rather than delirium or depression?

a.   Acute onset of symptoms
b.   Difficulty with concentration
c.   Signs of psychomotor slowing
d.   Good effort with testing, but wrong answers
e.   Patient complaint of memory loss

415. You are caring for a 79-year-old woman with symptoms suggesting Alzheimer disease. Which of the following clinical features of Alzheimer disease is most likely to remain intact until the late stages of the disease?

a.   The ability to recall new information
b.   The amount of conversational output
c.   The ability to draw complex figures (intersecting boxes or a clock)
d.   The ability to calculate (balance a checkbook)
e.   Appropriate social behavior

416. The daughter of one of your patients accompanies her mother to the office to discuss her concerns. The mother seems to have had progressive cognitive failure over the last year. According to the daughter, she loses function in a stepwise fashion. She seems to stabilize, but suddenly becomes less able to remember things or care for herself. This has happened several times in the last year. Given this history, which of the following is the likely etiology of her dementia?

a. Alzheimer disease
b. Parkinson disease
c. Alcoholic dementia
d. Vascular dementia
e. Depression

417. You decide to treat a 72-year-old man for Alzheimer dementia. You choose to use donepezil (Aricept), and begin therapy. With respect to disease progression, which of the following statements best describes donepezil's effect on Alzheimer dementia?

a. It dramatically slows the progression of neurodegeneration
b. It modestly slows the progression of neurodegeneration
c. It has no effect on the progression of neurodegeneration
d. It modestly increases the progression of neurodegeneration
e. It dramatically increases the progression of neurodegeneration

418. You are treating a patient with the classic signs of dementia. His caretaker reports that he has been having complex visual hallucinations and a tremor. On examination, he appears to have masked facies, has a slight tremor, and a shuffling gait. His cognitive decline is stable and present. Which of the following medications should be avoided in this case?

a. Cholinesterase inhibitors
b. SSRI
c. Tricyclic antidepressants
d. Antipsychotics
e. Benzodiazepines

419. You are caring for a patient who appears to have advanced Alzheimer dementia. Which of the following medications has been shown to result in statistically significant benefit in advanced cases of dementia?

a. Donepezil
b. Galantamine
c. Rivastigmine
d. Memantine
e. Ginkgo biloba

420. You are performing a screening physical examination on a 47-year-old man. He is generally healthy, and his review of systems is negative. His mother has type 2 diabetes, and he is overweight. Which of the following is generally accepted as the test of choice to screen for type 2 diabetes?

a. A random glucose test
b. A fasting glucose
c. A urinalysis to screen for glycosuria
d. A 1-hour glucose tolerance test
e. A 3-hour glucose tolerance test

421. You are evaluating a 36-year-old obese woman who complains of fatigue. She denies polydipsia, polyuria, polyphagia, or weight loss. Which of the following laboratory reports confirms the diagnosis of diabetes?

a. A random glucose reading of 221 mg/dL
b. A random glucose reading of 221 mg/dL, and another, on a later date, of 208 mg/dL
c. A fasting glucose measurement of 128 mg/dL
d. A glucose reading, taken 2 hours after a 75-g glucose load, of 163 mg/dL
e. A fasting glucose of 114 mg/dL, and a reading of 184 mg/dL 2 hours after a 75-g glucose load

422. An 18-year-old morbidly obese patient in your office is found to have a fasting glucose of 314 mg/dL. Which of the following test results indicates that he is a type 1 diabetic?

a. Low levels of C-peptide
b. Markedly elevated levels of C-peptide
c. Elevated levels of microalbumin in the urine
d. A markedly elevated hemoglobin A1C
e. Nerve conduction studies showing mild peripheral neuropathy

423. You are managing a 36-year-old woman with a new diagnosis of type 2 diabetes. Her hemoglobin A1C was 7.2% at diagnosis. Her subsequent sugars were well-controlled using metformin, 1000 mg twice daily. At her visit 3 months later, her blood pressure is 100/72 mm Hg, her hemoglobin A1C was 6.0%, but her microalbumin screen is positive. Which of the following is the most appropriate response?

a. Continue weight loss and recheck in 3 months
b. Limit dietary protein intake
c. Intensify diabetic therapy to more tightly control glucose
d. Initiate therapy with an ACE inhibitor
e. Refer to nephrology

424. A 44-year-old man is seeing you for a routine diabetic check. He was diagnosed with type 2 diabetes 2 years ago. He is worried because his grandmother went blind as a complication from her diabetes. Which of the following statements about diabetic retinopathy is true?

a. The risk of retinopathy increases with increased hemoglobin A1C levels.
b. It generally takes 10 to 20 years to see signs of retinopathy in a diabetic patient.
c. A daily aspirin decreases the risk of retinopathy development.
d. The first sign of retinopathy is usually the growth of new vessels on the retina.
e. Retinopathy is an uncommon cause of visual loss in this day and age.

425. You are seeing an African American man with newly diagnosed diabetes. His blood pressure at the last visit was 148/86 mm Hg, and at this visit it is 142/90 mm Hg. What should your first choice for blood pressure control be?

a. A β-blocker
b. A thiazide diuretic
c. An ACE inhibitor
d. A calcium channel blocker
e. An α-blocker

426. You are following a type 2 diabetic woman in her 50s. Six months ago, you checked her lipid profile. At that time, her total cholesterol was 245 mg/dL, her low-density lipoprotein (LDL) was 148 mg/dL, her high-density lipoprotein (HDL) was 30 mg/dL, and her triglycerides were 362. She has tried lifestyle modifications, but despite losing weight and exercising, her profile hasn't substantially changed. Which of the following is the first-line treatment for this patient?

a. Continued lifestyle modifications
b. A 3-hydroxy-3-methylglutaryl-CoA (HMG-CoA) [P1] reductase inhibitor (a "statin")
c. Niacin
d. Fibric acid derivatives
e. Bile acid resin

427. A 39-year old diabetic man asks you questions about his diet. Which of the following is true?

a. A high-fiber diet improves glycemic control
b. A low-carbohydrate diet improves glycemic control
c. A high-protein diet improves glycemic control
d. Sucrose should not be included in the diabetic diet
e. A formalized dietary program is more likely to produce long-term sustained effects

428. A 44-year-old African American with type 2 diabetes transfers care to you. Reviewing her records, you find she is on the maximum dose of sulfonylurea, but her hemoglobin A1C is 9.2% (H). Review of her baseline laboratory tests reveals normal liver enzymes and a creatinine of 2.3 mg/dL. Which of the following management options would be most beneficial?

a. Change to another sulfonylurea
b. Add a biguanide
c. Add a meglitinide
d. Add a thiazolidinedione
e. Add an α-glucosidase inhibitor

429. A 48-year-old woman has been treated for type 2 diabetes for 6 years with metformin 2000 mg daily, and glyburide 10 mg daily. She is modestly compliant with her diet, medications, and exercise. She is 69-in tall and weighs 278 lb. Her most recent HbA$_{1C}$ is 8.2% which has been relatively unchanged over the past 18 months. If weight loss is a therapeutic priority for this patient, which of the following would represent a logical next step?

a. Increase her glyburide to the maximum dose of 10 mg twice daily
b. Add a long-acting, basal insulin such as insulin glargine, discontinue glyburide, and maintain metformin
c. Add an insulin sensitizing agent such as pioglitazone or rosiglitazone to her regimen
d. Add an incretin-mimetic such as exenatide to her regimen
e. Simplify the regimen by discontinuing all oral medications and substituting a long-acting basal insulin plus a rapid-acting preprandial insulin such as insulin aspart

430. You have been treating a 46-year-old woman for type 2 diabetes for 2 years with metformin 2000 mg daily. She is compliant with her diet and medications, and exercises regularly. She is 65-in tall and weighs 200 lb. Her most recent HbA$_{1C}$ is 8.0% which is elevated from 7.8% 3 months ago. You added the insulin-sensitizing agent rosiglitazone to her regimen 2 weeks ago. The patient presents today complaining of a problem that she attributes to the new medication. Which of the following is the most likely complaint?

a. Symptomatic hypoglycemia
b. Edema and weight gain
c. Cough
d. Paradoxical hyperglycemia
e. GI intolerance

431. A 48-year-old man with type 2 diabetes returns for a follow-up appointment. He currently takes glipizide, pioglitazone, and acarbose, and wants to know more about sitagliptin (Januvia). Which of the following best explains its mechanism of action?

a. Inhibition of glucagon release
b. Increases the sensitivity of the body to insulin
c. Inhibition of hepatic gluconeogenesis
d. Inhibition of gastric emptying
e. Suppression of glucagon elaboration and delayed gastric emptying

432. You are thinking about starting a type 2 diabetic on insulin therapy to improve her glucose control. Which of the following insulin types has the most rapid onset of action?

a. Aspart (Novolog)
b. Regular
c. Lente
d. Ultralente
e. Glargine (Lantus)

433. You are thinking about starting a type 2 diabetic on insulin therapy to improve her glucose control. Which of the following insulin preparations has a peak or maximum action at approximately 5 hours?

a. Aspart (Novolog)
b. Regular
c. Lente
d. Ultralente
e. Glargine (Lantus)

434. You are thinking about starting a type 2 diabetic on insulin therapy to improve her glucose control. Which of the following insulin preparations has the longest duration of action?

a. Aspart (Novolog)
b. Regular
c. Lente
d. Ultralente
e. Glargine (Lantus)

435. After a period of noncompliance, one of your type 1 diabetics has been hospitalized for diabetic ketoacidosis. He has required approximately 100 U of insulin in a 24-hour period in the hospital using a sliding scale. You decide to begin split-dose therapy with neutral protamine Hagedorn (NPH) and regular insulin. How much NPH insulin should be given to this patient in the morning?

a. 25 U
b. 33 U
c. 50 U
d. 66 U
e. 75 U

436. You are caring for a type 1 diabetic who has been hospitalized with diabetic ketoacidosis, and determining an appropriate insulin regimen for her. She has required 60 U of insulin per day to maintain adequate control in the hospital. You decide to use insulin glargine (Lantus) and aspart (Lispro) in combination. What should her Lantus dose be?

a. 10 U
b. 20 U
c. 30 U
d. 40 U
e. 50 U

437. You have maximized oral therapy for a type 2 diabetic in your office. She works hard at diet and exercise, and is on maximal doses of oral hypo-glycemics, but her glycosolated hemoglobin is 8.6%. You decide to add insulin to her regimen. She is currently 67 in tall and weighs 100 kg. How much NPH should you give her at night as an addition to her current regimen?

a. 5 U
b. 10 U
c. 15 U
d. 20 U
e. 25 U

438. A 62-year-old woman sees you for preoperative clearance for a right hip replacement. Her past medical history is significant for hypertension, chronic kidney disease, osteoarthritis, and type 2 diabetes. During your examination, you detect a painless mass in her lower right abdomen. You schecule a CT scan with angiographic contrast. Which one of this patients' medications should be held prior to her receiving radiocontrast dye?

a. Metoprolol XL 100 mg
b. Metformin ER 1000 mg
c. Lisinopril 20 mg
d. Aspirin 325 mg
e. Pentoxifylline 400 mg

✓ **439.** You are caring for a 26-year-old man with dyslipidemia and a family history of early coronary arterial disease. Laboratory analysis reveals a low HDL. Which of the following interventions, if adopted by the patient, would raise his HDL levels to the greatest extent?

a. Use alcohol in moderation
b. Lose weight
c. Increase dietary intake of protein
d. Decrease dietary intake of cholesterol
e. Reduce life stress

440. You have performed a screening lipid profile on an otherwise healthy man. His results indicate elevated triglycerides, a low HDL, a high LDL, an elevated total cholesterol, and an elevated very low-density lipoprotein (VLDL). You'd like to rescreen him in the fasting state. Which of the following laboratory values is likely to decrease in the fasting state?

a. Serum triglycerides
b. HDL
c. LDL
d. Total cholesterol
e. VLDL

✓ **441.** You did screening cholesterol tests on a 35-year-old man and found his results to be:

Total cholesterol:	220 mg/dL (H)
LDL:	125 mg/dL (H)
HDL:	34 mg/dL (L)
Triglycerides:	307 mg/dL (H)
C-reactive protein:	2.4 mg/dL (H)

Which of his laboratory results is the best predictor of an adverse outcome in this patient?

a. Total cholesterol
b. LDL
c. HDL
d. Triglycerides
e. C-reactive protein

442. Through counseling and education, you have convinced a 35-year-old man with dyslipidemia to quit smoking. If he remains a nonsmoker, how would you expect his lipid profile to change?

a. His total cholesterol will decrease
b. His LDL will decrease
c. His fasting triglycerides will decrease
d. His HDL will increase
e. His VLDL will decrease

443. You have prescribed niacin for a patient with elevated LDL and triglycerides. He reports nonadherence to this regimen because of significant flushing that occurs when he takes the medication. What would you recommend to avoid this side effect?

a. Take the niacin at night
b. Take the niacin with food
c. Take the niacin with milk
d. Take aspirin before taking the niacin
e. Take a proton pump inhibitor before taking the niacin

444. You are thinking about prescribing an HMG-CoA reductase inhibitor for a patient with dyslipidemia, but are concerned about medication interactions given the patient's other medical conditions. In order to avoid drug interactions, reduce his LDL and increase his HDL, which of the following medications is the best choice?

a. Atorvastatin
b. Simvastatin
c. Lovastatin
d. Pravastatin
e. Rosuvastatin

445. In an attempt to lower cholesterol through diet, you recommend that a 40-year-old male take fish oil. What is the lipid-lowering mechanism of action of fish oil?

a. Sequesters bile acids
b. Changes hepatic metabolism of lipoprotein
c. Inhibits HMG-CoA reductase
d. Interferes with cholesterol absorption in the gut
e. Decreases secretion of triglycerides by the liver

446. You are seeing a 28-year-old man with significantly elevated triglycerides. You are considering gemfibrozil (Lopid) therapy. What is the mechanism of action of gemfibrozil?

a. Sequesters bile acids
b. Changes hepatic metabolism of lipoprotein
c. Inhibits HMG-CoA reductase
d. Interferes with cholesterol absorption in the gut
e. Decreases secretions of triglycerides by the liver

447. You are working with a 44-year-old man with difficult to manage dyslipidemia. He is taking atorvastatin (Lipitor) at maximum dosages, and you are considering adding ezetemibe (Zetia) to improve the lipid profile. How does ezetemibe work to help lower cholesterol?

a. Sequestration of bile acids
b. Changing hepatic metabolism of lipoproteins
c. Inhibits HMG-CoA reductase
d. Interferes with cholesterol absorption in the gut
e. Decreases secretion of triglycerides by the liver

448. You are caring for a patient with a poor lipid profile. His HDL is low, his LDL is high, and his triglycerides are also high. Which of the following medications would have the most beneficial effect on his HDL?

a. Lovastatin
b. Colestipol
c. Ezetimibe
d. Fenofibrate
e. Cholestyramine

449. You are caring for a patient with a poor lipid profile. His HDL is low, his LDL is high, and his triglycerides are also high. Which of the following medications would have the most beneficial effect on his LDL?

a. Lovastatin
b. Colestipol
c. Ezetimibe
d. Fenofibrate
e. Cholestyramine

450. You are caring for a patient with a poor lipid profile. His HDL is low, his LDL is high, and his triglycerides are also high. Which of the following medications would have the most beneficial effect on his triglycerides?

a. Lovastatin
b. Colestipol
c. Ezetimibe
d. Fenofibrate
e. Cholestyramine

451. You are treating a patient who is interested in more "natural" methods to control his cholesterol. He wants to use niacin. Which of the following statements regarding niacin is true?

a. It substantially decreases LDL.
b. It substantially raises HDL.
c. It has no effect on triglycerides.
d. Its side effects generally prevent it from being used.
e. It can't be used in patients who have concurrent diabetes.

452. You are seeing an HIV-positive patient who presents to discuss his current HIV therapy. His viral load is increasing and his CD4 count is falling. While obtaining his blood sample, your medical assistant sustained a needle stick injury. What is the best course of action in this situation?

a. Immediately test the medical assistant for HIV antibodies and begin treatment if positive
b. Immediately test the medical assistant for HIV viral load and begin treatment if detectable
c. Immediately test the medical assistant for HIV antibodies and begin zidovudine therapy
d. Immediately test the medical assistant for HIV viral load and begin zidovudine therapy
e. Immediately test the medical assistant for HIV antibodies and begin at least two drug therapy

453. You are taking care of a 22-year-old woman with fever, aches, and fatigue. Her history reveals intravenous drug abuse, and you suspect acute HIV infection. Which of the following tests is best to rule out acute HIV?

a. Enzyme-linked immunosorbent assay (ELISA)
b. Western blot
c. Immunofluorescent antibody test
d. Quantitative plasma HIV RNA (viral load)
e. CD4 lymphocyte count

454. You are caring for an HIV-infected woman. She had a normal Pap test 2 weeks ago. Which of the following is true?

a. She needs a repeat Pap test in 6 months
b. She needs a repeat Pap test in 12 months
c. She needs a colposcopy
d. She needs to have a colposcopy instead of her next Pap test
e. She should have prophylactic cone biopsy of the cervix

455. You are caring for a 38-year-old woman with a long history of intra-venous drug abuse. She was diagnosed with HIV 2 years ago, and has been doing well on therapy without disease progression. You order a purified protein derivative skin test for tuberculosis (TB). What amount of induration indicates a positive test?

a. Any induration indicates a positive test
b. 3 mm
c. 5 mm
d. 10 mm
e. 15 mm

456. A 38-year-old HIV-positive man follows up in your office for routine care. Unfortunately, his antiretroviral therapy is failing, and his CD4 count is falling. At his last two visits, his CD4 count has been less than 65 lymphocytes/mm^3. Prophylaxis for which of the following should be instituted at this time?

a. *Mycobacterium avium* complex
b. Fungal infections
c. Herpes simplex
d. Herpes zoster
e. Cytomegalovirus

457. You are seeing a patient with a long-standing HIV infection. The patient has been unable to afford his medication regimen and has been off medication for several months. He presents with shortness of breath. Blood gasses obtained emergently reveal a PaO_2 of 65 mm Hg. His chest x-ray is shown below:

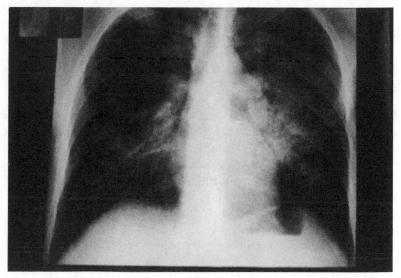

(Reproduced, with permission, from Knoop K, Stack L, Storrow A. Atlas of Emergency Medicine, 2nd ed. New York: McGraw-Hill, 2002: 666.)

Assuming the patient is not allergic, which of the following is the best first-line treatment?

a. Azithromycin
b. Trimethoprim-sulfamethoxazole
c. Trimethoprim-sulfamethoxazole and corticosteroids
d. Triple drug treatment against TB
e. Quadruple drug treatment against TB

√**458.** Which of the following patients should be tested for HIV-medication resistance as part of his or her workup?

a. A patient newly diagnosed with HIV with an undetectable viral load
b. A patient who was diagnosed with HIV 5 years ago, currently with an undetectable viral load without medication treatment
c. A patient who was diagnosed with HIV 5 years ago, currently with an undetectable viral load on medication therapy
d. A person who was diagnosed with HIV 10 years ago, currently with an undetectable viral load without medication treatment
e. A person who was diagnosed with HIV 10 years ago, currently with an undetectable viral load on triple therapy

√**459.** You have seen a 36-year-old man with elevated blood pressure. On one occasion, his blood pressure was 163/90 mm Hg, and on a second occasion, his blood pressure was 158/102 mm Hg. You have encouraged lifestyle modifications including weight loss using exercise and dietary changes. Despite some modest weight loss, at his current visit, his blood pressure is 166/92 mm Hg. Which of the following is the best treatment strategy at this point?

a. Use a thiazide diuretic
b. Use an ACE inhibitor
c. Use an angiotensin receptor blocker
d. Use a β-blocker
e. Use a two drug combination of medications

√**460.** You are examining a 40-year-old patient for the first time, and find her blood pressure to be 155/92 mm Hg. Which of the following physical examination findings, if present, would indicate a secondary cause of hypertension?

a. Left-sided carotid bruit
b. Distended jugular veins
c. Precordial heave
d. Absence of a femoral pulse
e. Papilledema

461. You have just diagnosed a 35-year-old man with hypertension. He is otherwise healthy and has no complaints. Which of the following is indicated in the initial evaluation?

a. TSH level assessment
b. Resting electrocardiogram
c. Stress test
d. Echocardiogram
e. Renal ultrasound

462. You are treating a 61-year-old man for hypertension. He is not responding well to combination therapy with a thiazide diuretic and a β-blocker. On physical examination, you note an abdominal bruit. Which of the following tests is most likely to help you evaluate him further?

a. Chest x-ray
b. Captopril renal scan
c. Urinary metanephrines and vanillymandelic acid levels
d. Aortic CT scan
e. Echocardiogram

463. You are counseling a 33-year-old obese woman with hypertension. Which of the following interventions would lower her systolic blood pressure the most?

a. Weight loss amounting to 10 kg
b. Adopting a diet high in fruits, vegetables, and low-fat dairy products
c. Restricting dietary sodium
d. Increasing physical activity at least 30 minutes a day, most days of the week
e. Limit alcohol consumption to no more than 1 drink per day

464. Despite lifestyle changes, a 37-year-old patient of yours still has blood pressures above goal. She has no other medical concerns, and no abnormalities on physical examination or initial laboratory evaluation. Which of the following medications is best as an initial first-line monotherapy?

a. A thiazide diuretic
b. An ACE inhibitor
c. An angiotensin receptor blocker
d. A calcium channel blocker
e. A β-blocker

465. A 48-year-old male patient suffered from a stroke. After full recovery, he follows up at your office. Which of the following medication options has been proven to lower his blood pressure and prevent recurrent stroke?

a. An ACE inhibitor
b. Hydrochlorothiazide
c. An ACE inhibitor and hydrochlorothiazide
d. A β-blocker
e. A β-blocker and hydrochlorothiazide

466. A 55-year-old man comes to your office after not being seen by a physician in more than 10 years. He is found to be hypertensive, and his creatinine is found to be 2.3 mg/dL (H). Which medication is most likely to control his blood pressure and decrease the likelihood of progression of his renal disease?

a. A thiazide diuretic
b. An ACE inhibitor
c. A calcium channel blocker
d. A β-blocker
e. An aldosterone antagonist

467. You have diagnosed a 35-year-old African American man with hypertension. Lifestyle modifications helped reduce his blood pressure, but he was still above goal. You chose to start hydrochlorothiazide, 25 mg daily. This helped his blood pressure, but it is still 142/94 mm Hg. Which of the following is the best approach to take in this situation?

a. Increase her hydrochlorothiazide to 50 mg/d
b. Change to a loop diuretic
c. Change to an ACE inhibitor
d. Change to a β-blocker
e. Add an ACE inhibitor

468. You are seeing a 49-year-old man with a known history of hypercholesterolemia and hypertension who has had recent complaints of chest pain. He reports a chest pressure, described as "heaviness" in the substernal area. It is not associated with activity, but will occur intermittently throughout the day. Which of the following is the best way to describe what the patient is feeling?

a. Classic angina
b. Atypical angina
c. Anginal equivalent
d. Nonanginal pain
e. Atypical nonanginal pain

469. You are seeing a 36-year-old man complaining of shortness of breath. He reports symptoms associated with activity and relieved by rest. He is otherwise healthy, takes no medications, and denies chest pain or pressure. Which of the following is the best way to describe what the patient is feeling?

a. Classic angina
b. Atypical angina
c. Anginal equivalent
d. Nonanginal pain
e. Atypical nonanginal pain

470. You are seeing a 44-year-old woman with a known history of asthma who has had recent complaints of chest pain. She reports a stabbing pain that seems to be worse with inspiration. It is not associated with activity, but will occur intermittently throughout the day. Which of the following is the best way to describe what the patient is feeling?

a. Classic angina
b. Atypical angina
c. Anginal equivalent
d. Nonanginal pain
e. Atypical nonanginal pain

471. You are evaluating a 39-year-old otherwise healthy man with a family history of ischemic heart disease. He describes chest pressure that radiates to his jaw when he walks up steps at work. You order an ECG in the office, shown below:

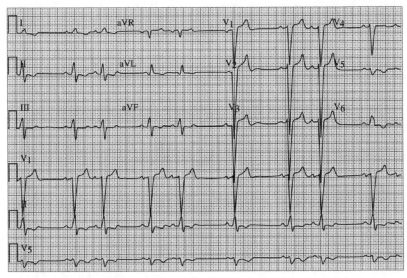

(Reproduced, with permission, from Ferry D. Basic Electrocardiography in Ten Days, 1st ed. New York: McGraw-Hill, 2001: 83.)

Which of the following is the test of choice to determine if his chest pain is because of cardiac ischemia?

a. Exercise treadmill test
b. Thallium exercise treadmill test
c. Stress echocardiogram
d. Persantine/thallium test
e. Dobutamine echocardiogram

472. You are caring for a 56-year-old man who presents to you for an evaluation of chest pain. You determine that an exercise treadmill test is necessary. The patient completes stage III of a Bruce protocol, achieves a heart rate of 136 beats per minute, and has an ST-segment depression of 1 mm in the three inferior leads at a heart rate of 130 beats per minute. These changes lasted 2 minutes into recovery. Which of the following features is a poor prognostic sign for the patient?

a. Being unable to reach stage IV of a Bruce protocol
b. Failure to achieve a heart rate of 140 beats per minute
c. Onset of ST-segment depression at a heart rate of 130 beats per minute
d. Having ST-segment depression in multiple leads
e. Having ST-segment depression lasting two minutes into recovery

473. You are medically treating an 85-year-old woman with stable angina, and choose to use nitrates. Which of the following is the most important consideration when using this medication?

a. Headache
b. Fatigue
c. Interactions with β-blockers
d. Interactions with calcium channel blockers
e. Development of tolerance

474. You have chosen to treat a 70-year-old man with ischemic heart disease using a β-blocker. Which of the following is the most appropriate endpoint for the use of β-blockers in this case?

a. Use no more than the equivalent of 40 mg twice daily of propranolol
b. Use the amount necessary to achieve a blood pressure of 100/70 mm Hg or less
c. Use the amount necessary to keep the heart rate between 50 to 60 beats per minute
d. Increase the dosage until fatigue limits use
e. Increase the amount until angina disappears

475. A 28-year-old man presents to your office to discuss weight management. You determine his body mass index (BMI) to be 28.2 kg/m². How should you classify this patient?

a. His BMI classifies him as being underweight
b. His BMI places him within the normal range
c. His BMI classifies him as being overweight
d. His BMI classifies him as obese
e. His BMI classifies him as morbidly obese

476. A 33-year-old woman is seeing you for weight management. At 5 ft 6 in tall and 230 lb, she reports a history of having difficulty with weight since her teenage years. The rest of her medical history is unremarkable. Using conventional dietary techniques, what is her chance of losing 20 lb and maintaining that weight loss for 2 years?

a. 1%
b. 5%
c. 10%
d. 20%
e. 50%

477. You are discussing weight management with an overweight 33-year-old woman. She has tried for years to lose weight, but despite multiple attempts, remains overweight. Which of the following is indicated in the workup of her weight concerns?

a. History and physical alone
b. CBC
c. TSH
d. Serum electrolytes
e. Luteinizing hormone to follicle-stimulating hormone ratio

478. You are working with an obese patient to help him lose weight. You are considering the use of orlistat (Xenical, Alli) to help the patient with weight reduction. Which of the following is the mechanism of action for this medication?

a. It is an appetite suppressant.
b. It blocks the uptake of both serotonin and norepinephrine in the central nervous system.
c. It is a selective cannabinoid-1 receptor antagonist.
d. It reduces fat absorption in the GI tract.
e. It is a catecholaminergic amphetamine.

479. You are evaluating a patient whose BMI is 44 kg/m². You'd like the patient to consider weight-loss surgery, specifically a Roux-en-Y gastric bypass. Which of the following is true regarding this procedure?

a. The operative mortality rate for this procedure in the first 30 days is near 5%.
b. Complications from this procedure occur in approximately 40% of the cases.
c. The procedure can be expected to help the patient lose up to 30% of initial body weight.
d. Nutritional deficiencies after surgery are rare.
e. This surgery is reserved for people with BMI greater than 30 kg/m².

✓**480.** A 49-year-old African American perimenopausal woman is seeing you after having fractured her wrist. Her past medical history is significant for oral contraceptive use for 20 years, obesity, and Graves disease leading to current hypothyroidism. She nursed two children for 6 months each. Which component of the patient's history puts her at increased risk for osteoporosis?

a. African American race
b. Oral contraceptive use
c. Obesity
d. Graves disease
e. Breast-feeding

✓**481.** A 32-year-old woman is seeing you because her mother has been diagnosed with osteoporosis. She asks you what type of exercise will help her prevent the development of the disease. According to recommendations, which of the following exercises is most appropriate to help her maintain bone mass?

a. Tennis
b. Swimming
c. Cycling
d. Skating
e. Skiing

482. You are caring for a 48-year-old Caucasian woman with a history of anorexia nervosa in her late 20s. She was an elite track and field athlete in her late teens and early 20s, and was considered for the US Olympic team in her prime. Which of the following options is best for primary osteoporosis screening in this woman?

a. History
b. Physical examination
c. Serum calcium
d. Serum human osteocalcin levels
e. Bone density imaging

483. You are evaluating a 76-year-old woman on long-term glucocorticosteroid therapy for polymyalgia rheumatica. Which of the following is the diagnostic imaging test of choice to diagnose osteoporosis?

a. Plain radiographs
b. Single photon absorptiometry
c. Dual photon absorptiometry
d. DEXA scan
e. Quantitative CT of bone

484. You screened a 52-year-old, at-risk woman for osteoporosis using a DEXA scan. You received a T-score and a Z-score in the report. Which of the following indicates osteoporosis?

a. Equal T- and Z-score
b. T-score of +2.5
c. T-score of −2.5
d. Z-score of +2.5
e. Z-score of −2.5

485. You have diagnosed a 53-year-old woman with osteoporosis. She is postmenopausal, and you are considering estrogen-replacement therapy. Which of the following is a relative contraindication to estrogen-replacement therapy?

a. A history of breast cancer
b. A history of uterine cancer
c. A history of estrogen-dependent neoplasia
d. An abnormal genital bleeding
e. A history of a thromboembolic disorder

486. You are treating an elderly postmenopausal woman with osteoporosis. She recently suffered an acute osteoporotic vertebral fracture, and is suffering from secondary pain. Which of the following osteoporosis treatments also has analgesic effects with respect to bone pain?

a. Estrogen
b. Combination of calcium and vitamin D
c. Calcitonin
d. Alendronate (Fosamax)
e. Raloxifene (Evista)

487. You have just diagnosed osteoporosis in a postmenopausal woman. She is considering treatment alternatives and wonders about the bisphosphonates. Which of the following is the best description of how this class of medications works?

a. They increase calcium absorption in the GI tract
b. They block the activity of the cytokines that stimulate bone reabsorption
c. They bind to bone surfaces to inhibit osteoclast activity
d. They stimulate osteoblasts and increase bone formation
e. They mimic estrogen's effect on bone

488. You are seeing a 32-year-old woman for fatigue. Your differential diagnosis includes major depressive disorder, but she does not describe a depressed or irritable mood. Which of the following symptoms of depression must be present in order to diagnose a major depressive disorder in someone without depressed mood?

a. Sleep changes
b. Loss of interest or pleasure in usually enjoyable activities
c. Guilt or feelings of worthlessness
d. Loss of energy
e. Change in appetite

489. You are caring for a patient in your practice who has a problem with alcohol abuse. Upon direct questioning, he says that he drinks because he continually recounts stressful memories from being in the Iraq war. Which of the following medications is the best choice to treat his disorder?

a. Bupropion
b. Sertraline
c. Alprazolam
d. Valproic acid
e. Venlafaxine

490. You are discussing treatment options for a 43-year-old woman with major depressive disorder. Which of the following is a true statement regarding the effectiveness of treatment for depressive disorders?

a. Only about 25% of patients that receive medication alone will find the medication to be effective.
b. Patients who find one medication ineffective are likely to find all medications ineffective.
c. In order to prevent a relapse of depressive symptoms, patients should continue treatment for 3 to 4 months.
d. In general, patients respond best to the combination of medication and counseling.
e. Electroconvulsive therapy (ECT) is ineffective when compared with newer medical therapy.

491. You are treating a 48-year-old man for major depression. His medical history includes a head injury several years ago that has left him with a seizure disorder. Which of the following antidepressants would be contraindicated?

a. Venlafaxine
b. Nefazodone
c. Mirtazapine
d. Fluoxetine
e. Bupropion

492. Which of the following conditions is considered an anxiety disorder?

a. Obsessive-compulsive disorder
b. Conversion disorder
c. Somatization disorder
d. Anorexia nervosa
e. Histrionic personality disorder

493. You are following a 16-year-old girl with a suspected eating disorder. Which of the following, if present, would help differentiate anorexia nervosa from bulimia nervosa?

a. Binge eating or purging
b. The use of laxatives, diuretics, or enemas
c. Self-evaluation is unduly influenced by body weight and shape
d. Episodic lack of control over eating
e. Inappropriate behaviors to prevent weight gain

√ **494.** You decide to treat a severely depressed patient with fluoxetine. The response is dramatic, and on follow up he reports that he feels great. He's got a lot of energy—in fact he hasn't slept in 2 days. He just bought a new car despite losing his job. You suspect acute mania. Which of the following is the best choice of medications to control the acute symptoms?

a. Neuroleptics
b. Lithium
c. Valproic acid
d. Carbamazepine
e. Lamotrigine

√ **495.** A 26-year-old male college graduate is seeing you for an office visit. He is concerned that he may have adult attention deficit hyperactivity disorder (ADHD). Which of the following is true regarding this condition?

a. The symptoms are likely to be more pronounced in adults as compared with children.
b. Children diagnosed with ADHD commonly continue to have symptoms into adulthood.
c. Sleep disturbance is a distinctive feature of adult ADHD.
d. Appetite disturbance is a distinctive feature of adult ADHD.
e. The symptom picture of adult ADHD mimics that in children.

496. What is the principal mechanism by which stimulant medications work to improve symptoms of ADHD?

a. Inhibition of serotonin reuptake
b. Stimulation of serotonin production
c. Inhibition of dopamine and norepinephrine reuptake
d. Stimulation of dopamine and norepinepherine production
e. Blocking the release of serotonin

√ **497.** A 45-year-old woman presents to your office for evaluation. She reports that over the last few weeks, she's noted an enlarging mass in the front of her neck. She feels well, has had no changes in her health, and denies symptoms of hyper- or hypothyroidism. She also denies recent viral illness. On examination, you note a diffusely enlarged thyroid that is tender to touch. Which of the following is her most likely diagnosis?

a. Hashimoto thyroiditis
b. Subacute lymphocytic thyroiditis
c. Subacute granulomatous thyroiditis
d. Suppurative thyroiditis
e. Invasive fibrous thyroiditis

498. A 26-year-old woman presents with weight gain, lethargy, dry skin, sweatiness, cold intolerance, and thinning hair. You suspect hypothyroidism and order the appropriate laboratory tests. Her TSH is high, and her free T_3 and free T_4 are both low. Which of the following is the most likely diagnosis?

a. Primary hypothyroidism
b. Secondary hypothyroidism
c. Iodine deficiency
d. Thyroid hormone resistance
e. Subclinical hypothyroidism

499. You are screening a 35-year-old woman who presents with tachycardia, nervousness, tremor, palpitations, heat intolerance, and weight loss. You suspect Graves disease. What single test is best for differentiating Graves disease from other causes of hyperthyroidism?

a. TSH
b. TSH with free T_4 and free T_3
c. Thyroid receptor antibodies
d. Radionucleotide imaging of the thyroid
e. Thyroid ultrasound

500. When examining a 35-year-old, you notice a firm 3-cm thyroid nodule. His thyroid studies are normal, and he is clinically euthyroid. Radionucleotide imaging demonstrates uptake in the thyroid nodule. Which of the following is the most likely diagnosis?

a. Colloid cyst
b. Thyroid adenoma
c. Thyroid carcinoma
d. Metastatic disease
e. Neurofibroma

Chronic Conditions

Answers

338. The answer is d. (*South-Paul, pp 182-189.*) The sexual response is divided into four phases. The first is libido (or desire/interest). This phase requires androgens and an intact sensory system. The second phase is arousal (or excitement) and in men, involves erection. Vascular arterial or inflow problems are by far the most common cause, though mood disorders, stressors, and alcohol abuse may all play a role. Lack of attraction to a partner would represent a disorder of desire, not arousal.

339. The answer is b. (*South-Paul, pp 182-189.*) In patients with decreased sex drive, laboratory workup should be directed by the history and physical examination findings. In a patient with no other complaints and no physical examination findings, assessment of hormone status is indicated. Testosterone levels should be checked in the morning, when they peak. Free testosterone is a more accurate measure of androgen status, as it is a measure of bioavailable testosterone. The TSH and prolactin levels may be indicated in the presence of other complaints or physical findings. PSA would not be helpful.

340. The answer is e. (*South-Paul, pp 182-189.*) Many medications can cause sexual dysfunction. Medications that commonly cause ejaculatory dysfunction in men include β-blockers, α-blockers, antipsychotics, and SSRIs. Hydrochlorothiazide can cause erectile dysfunction and decreased libido. Omeprazole and bupropion often do not negatively impact sexual functioning.

341. The answer is e. (*South-Paul, pp 182-189.*) Tricyclics and SSRIs frequently cause sexual dysfunction. Bupropion actually decreases the orgasm threshold and is least likely to cause sexual dysfunction.

342. The answer is b. (*South-Paul, pp 182-189.*) Premature ejaculation is the most common sexual dysfunction in men, affecting about 29% of the general population. Alprostadil is used for erectile dysfunction, but would not positively effect premature ejaculation. Fluoxetine raises the threshold for orgasm, making it an effective treatment option. Bupropion and silendafil may decrease the orgasmic threshold and might be problematic. Atenolol may cause erectile dysfunction, but would likely not treat premature ejaculation.

343. The answer is d. *(South Paul, pp 182-189.)* Oral testosterone replacement is not recommended because of a prominent first-pass effect and potential for significant liver damage. Intramuscular injections are associated with fluctuations in blood levels. Transdermal preparations offer the benefit of consistency in therapeutic levels, but patches may produce local skin reactions. Gel offers transdermal absorption, but does not cause the local skin reactions of patches. Sublingual testosterone is not used in men.

344. The answer is b. *(Mengel, pp 593-603.)* Characteristics known to influence the epidemiology of substance use disorders include gender (men are more likely to be affected than women), age (disorders become less frequent with age), marital status (single persons have a higher risk than married), employment (the unemployed are at higher risk), and level of education (less educated persons are at higher risk). Though one would expect job stress to influence substance use, studies have not shown this to be true.

345. The answer is c. *(Mengel, pp 593-603.)* Most clinicians agree that psychiatric disorders cannot be reliably assessed in patients who are currently or recently intoxicated. Alcohol is a depressant, and may be the main factor in the patient's depressive symptoms. Detoxification and a period of abstinence are necessary before an evaluation for other psychiatric disorders can be effectively completed.

346. The answer is d. *(Mengel, pp 593-603.)* Most people who abuse alcohol have completely normal laboratory studies. However, of the tests listed in the question, the GGT is the most sensitive. Elevated GGT is shown to be more sensitive than an elevated MCV, ALT, AST, or LDH. The specificity of the GGT is low, however, being elevated in nonalcoholic liver disease, diabetes, pancreatitis, hyperthyroidism, heart failure, and anticonvulsant use.

347. The answer is a. *(South-Paul pp 614-625.)* An elevated MCV is 96% specific for alcohol abuse with a 63% predictive value. The GGT is 76% specific with a predictive value of 61%. AST, ALT, and LDH are less specific and have a worse predictive value.

348. The answer is b. *(Mengel, pp 593-603.)* Drugs used for addiction work in one of four ways. They either cause the body to have a negative reaction to an ingested drug, reduce the reinforcing effects of an ingested drug, block the effects of the drug by binding to the receptor site, or saturate the receptor sites with agonists that do not create the drug's desired effect. Naltrexone is known to be helpful for both opiate addiction and alcohol addiction. Naltrexone saturates opiate receptor sites and leaves them unavailable for opiate attachment. For alcohol abuse, naltrexone works differently, reducing the reinforcing effect of alcohol (not allowing patients to become "drunk").

349. The answer is a. *(Mengel, pp 593-603.)* Disulfiram cause the body to have a negative reaction to ingested alcohol, regardless of the form. As such, it is a deterrent. The reaction to alcohol that occurs is manifested by flushing, nausea, and vomiting. Importantly, alcohol in cough medicines, mouthwashes, and other forms must be avoided, as the reaction does not discriminate based on from where the alcohol comes.

350. The answer is d. *(South-Paul pp 614-625.)* Disulfiram, naltrexone, SSRIs, and acamprosate are currently used to prevent relapse of alcoholism. Although the goal of abstinence cannot be met by medication alone, in selected patients, it may improve chances for recovery. Acamprosate seems to be the most effective of these medications. It effects both γ-aminobutyric acid (GABA) and glutamine neurotransmission, both of which are important in alcohol's effect on the brain. The effects of this medication appear to be greater and longer-lasting than naltrexone. The addition of disulfiram can increase the effectiveness of acamprosate alone.

351. The answer is b. *(Rakel, pp 1339-1345.)* The nicotine-withdrawal syndrome is a serious obstacle for patients wishing to stop smoking. Withdrawal symptoms often begin within hours after the last cigarette. Early abstinence is characterized by irritability, anxiety, restlessness, depressed mood, inattention, and insomnia. Nicotine replacement is often effective in lessening some of these symptoms, as is bupropion.

352. The answer is a. *(South-Paul pp 626-633.)* Nicotine-replacement therapy increases the chance that a smoker will quit. Using two forms of nicotine replacement, like a patch and a gum, allows a baseline level of nicotine to be in the patient's system and allows for a bolus during times of craving. This improves quit rates and is recommended if other forms of nicotine replacement are ineffective alone.

353. The answer is c. (*South-Paul pp 614-625.*) Varenicline is a selective nicotinic receptor partial agonist. There are no known drug interactions, and it is largely excreted in the urine. Dose modifications would be needed in people with severe renal disease. Common side effects include nausea, insomnia, and abnormal dreams. It is safe in persons with seizure disorders, though bupropion is not. Varenicline is taken for 1 week before the quit date, and therefore can be taken while a person is still smoking.

354. The answer is d. (*South-Paul pp 614-625.*) Behavioral intervention alone is an option for this patient, but you would at least double his success rate if you add medication to this. First-line therapies include nicotine replacement, bupropion, and varenicline. Nicotine replacement should be used with caution when working up unstable angina. His seizure disorder contraindicates the use of bupropion. Clonidine is not approved by the FDA for smoking cessation, but several studies have shown that it doubles the rate of abstinence. Clonidine represents a second-line therapy for those who have failed the first-line therapies.

355. The answer is c. (*Rakel, pp 1339-1345.*) Cocaine withdrawal does not produce a significant physiologic withdrawal. Intoxication with cocaine does produce elevated heart rate and blood pressure. The most common problem produced by cocaine withdrawal is known as a "crash." The crash is characterized by extreme fatigue and significant depression. Relapse is common during the crash because return to use provides quick and reliable relief.

356. The answer is c. (*Rakel, pp 1339-1345.*) Opiate withdrawal is well-characterized, and although not life-threatening in otherwise healthy adults, can cause severe discomfort. Symptoms from a short-acting drug like heroin can occur within just a few hours. Withdrawal from longer acting opiates may not cause symptoms for days. Early symptoms include lacrimation, rhinorrhea, yawning, and diaphoresis. Restlessness and irritability occur later, with bone pain, nausea, diarrhea, abdominal cramping, and mood lability occurring even later.

Cocaine does not have a significant physiologic withdrawal syndrome, but craving is intense. Marijuana-withdrawal syndrome is also not physiologically significant. Ecstasy can be considered a hallucinogen or a stimulant, and withdrawal is often associated with depression, but not the symptoms described above. Benzodiazepine withdrawal mimics alcohol withdrawal, and is associated with hypertension, tachycardia, and possibly seizures.

357. The answer is a. (*South-Paul, pp 233-248.*) The picture shown demonstrates Heberden nodes (at the distal interphalangeal joints) and Bouchard nodes (at the proximal interphalangeal joints). These abnormalities are commonly classified as osteoarthritis, but are only infrequently associated with pain or disability. Laboratory evaluation will only rarely show an inflammatory process, and an elevated uric acid level would be an incidental finding.

358. The answer is b. (*South-Paul, pp 233-248.*) Osteoarthritis is characterized as being pauciarticular. The pain is worse with activity and improved with rest. There is often mild swelling, but warmth and an effusion are rare. Crepitus is common, as is malalignment of the joint. RA tends to be polyarticular and symmetric. Morning stiffness improves with activity. Gout is abrupt in onset and monoarticular. Tendonitis and fibromyalgia are not associated with joint swelling and crepitus.

359. The answer is c. (*South-Paul, pp 233-248.*) The patient's history is consistent with an attack of gout. The most common presentation of gout is podagra (an abrupt, intense inflammation of the first MTP joint), but any joint can be affected. It is characterized by an abrupt onset of monoarticular symptoms with pain at rest and with movement. The attacks often occur overnight, after an inciting event (excessive alcohol or a heavy meal). The sufferer often cites exquisite pain, with even slight pressure on the joint being quite painful. Osteoarthritis and RA would not occur so abruptly. A stress fracture would likely not be as painful at rest, and cellulitis would generally not be as abrupt or painful.

Septic arthritis and gout may be clinically indistinguishable, unless the joint fluid is analyzed.

360. The answer is a. (*South-Paul, pp 233-248.*) RA is characterized by gradual, symmetric involvement of joints, with morning stiffness. Hands and feet are usually involved first, but it may spread to larger joints. Fatigue is a common complaint. On examination, symmetric swelling and tenderness are common, with associated rheumatoid nodules. Osteoarthritis is generally less symmetric and often occurs later in life. Gout is usually monoarticular. Tendonitis and fibromyalgia would be less likely to be associated with joint swelling.

361. The answer is e. (*South-Paul, pp 233-248.*) Oral steroids have a strong potential for ulcer formation, and although they may offer temporary relief, would not be indicated for chronic osteoarthritis. Another steroid injection would be of limited benefit, and most recommend no more than two injections per year to avoid hastening of the osteoarthritic process. Ketorolac is not indicated for intra-articular injection. Hyaluronic acid injections have been shown to provide symptomatic relief in osteoarthritis for up to 6 months, but given the malalignment demonstrated in his x-ray, knee replacement would likely be more beneficial. Indications for replacement include poorly controlled pain despite maximal therapy, malalignment, and decreased mobility or ambulation.

362. The answer is c. (*South-Paul, pp 233-248.*) Alcohol alters renal excretion of uric acid, allowing buildup of serum uric acid levels. This buildup allows crystals to precipitate in the joint spaces, causing the symptoms of gout.

363. The answer is d. (*South-Paul, pp 233-248.*) An evaluation of the joint aspirate is strongly recommended to establish the diagnosis of gout. It is critical to differentiate gout from infectious arthritis which is a medical emergency, and a joint aspirate will do this rapidly and accurately. The sedimentation rates and C-reactive protein are both nonspecific. Serum uric acid levels can be normal or high in the setting of acute gout. A 24-hour urine collection may help determine the most effective treatment for gout, but is not needed for diagnosis.

364. The answer is b. (*South-Paul, pp 233-248.*) The crystals typical of gout are needle-shaped and have negative birefringement. The crystals of pseudogout are rhomboid-shaped and demonstrate positive birefringement. Infectious arthritis, osteoarthritis, and RA would not present with crystals in the joint aspirate.

365. The answer is c. (*South-Paul, pp 233-248.*) Infectious arthritis, gout and pseudogout may all be associated with cloudy joint aspirate fluid. The aspirate fluid obtained from a gout or pseudogout flare may also have a WBC count of 50,000/mm^3 with a high proportion of PMN leukocytes. However, glucose levels fluid aspirated from a knee with gout or pseudogout would be normal.

366. The answer is d. (*South-Paul, pp 233-248.*) Fluid aspirated from an osteoarthritic knee is characterized by generally clear joint fluid with a WBC count of 2000/mm³ to 10,000/mm³. The distinguishing factor is the PMN leukocytes. In rheumatoid arthritis, more than 50% of the WBCs are PMNs, while in osteoarthritis, less than 50% of the WBCs are PMNs.

367. The answer is a. (*South-Paul, pp 233-248.*) While a short course of NSAID is one standard therapy for gout, another is a course of colchicine. Colchicine is given orally, one tablet every 1 to 2 hours until pain is controlled or side effects limit its use (the usual side effect is diarrhea). Most attacks respond to the first two or three pills, and the maximum number used in a 24-hour period is six. Corticosteroids can provide quick relief, but should be reserved if initial therapy fails. Opiates may control pain, but will not lead to resolution of the inflammation. Allopurinol and probenecid are effective treatments for prevention, but should be used cautiously, as they can precipitate a flare.

368. The answer is d. (*South-Paul, pp 233-248.*) Swelling of the proximal interphalangeal joints (shown here in the second and third fingers) is typical of RA. Symmetrical swelling is almost unique to RA, and even lupus, often confused with RA in the early stages, is rarely as consistently symmetrical. Fatigue is often out of proportion to the lack of sleep, and the prolonged morning stiffness in the history is essential to diagnosis.

369. The answer is a. (*South-Paul, pp 233-248.*) Extra-articular manifestations of RA can be seen at any stage of the disease. Most common are rheumatoid nodules that can occur anywhere on the body, but usually subcutaneously along pressure points. Vasculitis, dry eyes, dyspnea, or cough can all be seen. Cough and dyspnea may signal respiratory interstitial disease. Cardiac, GI, and renal systems are rarely involved. When a neuropathy is present, it is generally because of a compression syndrome, not as an extra-articular manifestation of the disease.

370. The answer is e. (*South-Paul, pp 233-248.*) In the past, most people treated the symptoms of RA with nonsteroidals until that was ineffective, then referred to rheumatology. Unfortunately, these agents did nothing to slow the progression of disease. The most important advancement in the treatment of RA has been the introduction of disease-modifying antirheumatic drugs (DMARDs). These agents not only control patient symptoms but suppress the underlying factors that result in synovitis, tissue reactivity, erosions, subluxations, and other complications. These should be managed by rheumatologists and started early to avoid or delay joint deformity.

371. The answer is b. (*McPhee, pp 204-216.*) Asthma is common, affecting approximately 5% of the population. While there is a genetic component to its development, the strongest identified predisposing factor for its development is atopy. Nonspecific predictors include upper respiratory infections, pneumonia, gastroesophageal reflux disease, and exposure to environmental smoke.

372. The answer is b. (*Rakel, pp 918-924.*) Environmental measures can be an important component of asthma control. They include keeping humidity in the home relatively low, under 50%, enclosing the mattress, box spring, and pillows with allergen impermeable covers (they can be dust reservoirs), laundering bed linens with hot water, and removing carpeting whenever possible. Air filters have not been shown to affect reservoir levels of house dust mite allergens.

373. The answer is a. (*Mengel, pp 415-423.*) The most important component in the diagnosis of asthma is history. Patients with asthma typically have recurrent episodes of wheezing, but not all asthma includes wheezing, and not all wheezing is asthma. Cough is the only symptom in cough-variant asthma. Allergy testing may help to identify specific allergens, but is not useful in diagnosing asthma. A chest x-ray is useful to rule-out other causes of cough or wheezing, but is not needed to diagnose asthma. Pulmonary function testing is usually confirmatory, not diagnostic. Provocative testing is indicated for the rare patient in whom the diagnosis is in question, but should be used cautiously, as life-threatening bronchospasm may occur.

374. The answer is c. (*South-Paul, pp 274-288.*) Asthma is classified by its severity, assessing daytime and nighttime symptoms. Patients with symptoms less than twice a week, with brief exacerbations, and with nighttime symptoms less than twice a month are classified as having "mild intermittent" asthma. There is no "moderate intermittent" classification. The "mild persistent" classification refers to symptoms more than twice a week but less than once a day, with symptoms that sometimes affect usual activity. Nighttime symptoms occur more than twice a month. The "moderate persistent" classification is characterized by daily symptoms and use of short-acting inhaler, with exacerbations that affect activity and may last for days. Nighttime symptoms occur at least weekly. "Severe persistent" asthma is characterized by continual symptoms that limit physical activities, with frequent exacerbations and nighttime symptoms.

375. The answer is d. (*South-Paul, pp 274-288.*) The patient described in this question fits the "moderate persistent" classification, characterized by daily symptoms and use of short-acting inhaler, with exacerbations that affect activity and may last for days. Nighttime symptoms occur at least weekly.

376. The answer is c. (*South-Paul, pp 274-288. Mengel, pp 415-423.*) Peak flow measurements parallel the FEV_1, and are an easy and inexpensive way to monitor asthma control. The peak flow "zone system" allows patients' to monitor their control and participate in the clinical decision-making around their illness. Measurements between 80% to 100% of the patient's personal best are in the "green zone," and indicate that the patient is doing well. Measurements between 50% to 80% of the personal best are in the "yellow zone," and are a warning to consider a step up in therapy (review of medication technique, adherence, and environmental control, or use additional medication). Measurements below 50% of the personal best are an indicator that the patient needs immediate medical attention.

377. The answer is c. (*Rakel, pp 918-924.*) Inhaled corticosteroids are the mainstay of long-term asthma treatment, and act at numerous sites in the inflammatory cascade. They should be prescribed for all patients except those with very mild asthma or contraindications. Changing short-acting agents would not likely be beneficial. Long-acting β-agonists do not impact airway inflammation and should not be used without a corticosteroid. A leukotriene receptor antagonist is an option, but is generally thought of as a "second best" choice. Inhaled corticosteroids and leukotriene antagonists have replaced cromolyn in current asthma therapy.

378. The answer is b. (*Rakel, pp 918-924.*) The patient described in this question has worsening asthma symptoms and needs additional therapy. Long-acting β-agonists are considered the most appropriate medication in this case, and are often packaged with an inhaled corticosteroid for ease of use. A leukotriene receptor antagonist would also be appropriate. A burst and taper of oral steroids may be appropriate for an acute flare, but not in this case. Cromolyn has associated compliance issues as it is dosed four times a day. Atrovent is usually not used unless there is a component of COPD, and theophylline, though an appropriate "third-line" agent, is not more effective than a long-acting β-agonist.

379. The answer is b. (*Rakel, pp 918-924.*) Long-acting β-agonists are less effective if not paired with inhaled corticosteroids. A leukotriene receptor antagonist is a better choice in this case. Cromolyn therapy has been replaced by newer agents, mainly because of compliance issues. Theophylline and oral steroids would not be indicated in this case.

380. The answer is a. (*Mengel, pp 273-277.*) Spondylolisthesis is an anterior displacement of vertebrae in relation to the one below. It is the most common cause of low back pain in patients younger than age 26, especially athletes. Back strain is also a common diagnosis, but would generally follow an inciting event, and pain would be associated with movement. The patient is likely too young for osteoarthritis to be a consideration, and a lumbar disk herniation can occur at any age, but is less likely to be the diagnosis in this case. Neoplasm is a rare cause of low back pain.

381. The answer is b. (*Mengel, pp 273-277.*) Back pain caused by an inflammatory condition (rheumatoid arthritis, ankylosing spondylitis, Reiter syndrome) are rare, but have characteristics that are helpful in differentiating them from other causes of pain. Inflammatory conditions generally produce greater pain and stiffness in the morning, while mechanical disorders tend to worsen throughout the day with activity. A disk herniation might be associated with radiation and neurological symptoms. A compression fracture would begin suddenly, and a neoplasm is unlikely to get better throughout the day.

382. The answer is c. (*Mengel, pp 273-277.*) The test described in this question is called the straight leg raising test. The test is considered positive when the patient feels pain below the knee when the leg is raised 30° to 60°. The positive test indicates nerve root irritation, likely because of a herniated disk. A back strain should not produce a positive straight leg raising test. A compression fracture may occur suddenly, but would be unlikely in an otherwise healthy young man. Neoplasms and inflammatory conditions would be less likely to occur suddenly.

383. The answer is b. (*Mengel, pp 273-277.*) MRI is indicated for people whose pain persists for more than 6 weeks despite normal radiographs and no response to conservative therapy. Flexion/extension films would not be helpful in identifying more concerning causes of pain. EMG is not indicated without neurological involvement. A bone scan and/or ESR should be considered in those with symptoms consistent with cancer or infection.

384. The answer is a. (*Mengel, pp 273-277.*) It is recommended that patients with low back pain maintain usual activities, as dictated by pain. Neither prolonged bed rest nor traction has been shown to be effective in returning people to their usual activities sooner. NSAIDs are effective for short-term symptomatic pain relief. Muscle relaxants appear to be effective as well. Opioids may be indicated in pain relief for those who have failed NSAIDs, but are significantly sedating. Steroids can be considered in those who have failed NSAID therapy.

385. The answer is b. (*Mengel, pp 295-300.*) The provocative maneuver described in this question is called Spurling test. It is positive with nerve root irritation that may accompany a disk herniation. It would not be positive with cervical strain, spondylosis (degenerative changes of the spinal vertebrae), or arthritis. Torticollis is a sudden onset of unilateral muscular pain, and would also not produce a positive Spurling test.

386. The answer is b. (*Mengel, pp 295-300.*) The Canadian cervical spine rules help to identify which patients with neck pain require radiographic evaluation. If a patient is unable to rotate his/her neck 45° regardless of pain, x-rays are indicated. MRI, bone scan, and DEXA scanning are not indicated in this situation.

387. The answer is b. (*Mengel, pp 429-441.*) Chronic bronchitis is defined as a productive cough lasting 3 consecutive months over 2 consecutive years. Emphysema is generally not a clinical diagnosis, requiring evidence of terminal airway airspace enlargement owing to alveoli destruction. Chronic bronchitis and emphysema are the clinical manifestations of COPD. Asthma is a result of airway hyperreactivity, and cannot be assumed given the above history. Bronchiectasis is a destruction of the bronchial walls leads to permanent dilation of the bronchi, with infection as the major cause. Clinical features include a persistent cough with purulent sputum production. Pneumonia would be unlikely given the clinical features described.

388. The answer is e. (*Mengel, pp 429-441.*) α_1-Antitrypsin deficiency is a rare genetic abnormality, accounting for less than 1% of the cases of COPD.

It should be suspected in people who develop COPD before age 50, especially in nonsmokers, and in people with a family history. The x-ray would show typical emphysematous blebs, especially in the basilar areas. HIV, CHF, and lung cancer are unlikely causes of the x-ray findings described. The patient does not meet the criteria for chronic bronchitis.

389. The answer is e. (*McPhee, pp 216-221.*) The single most important intervention in smokers with COPD is to encourage smoking cessation. However, the only drug therapy that has been shown to improve the natural history of COPD progression is supplemental oxygen in those patients that are hypoxemic. Bronchodilators do not alter the course of the decline in function, and COPD is generally not a steroid responsive disease. Antibiotics can be useful to treat infection and exacerbation, but no convincing evidence exists to support their use chronically.

390. The answer is e. (*Mengel, pp 429-441.*) The patient described in the question has risk factors and physical stigmata of COPD. Office spirometry is helpful to diagnose COPD and assess its severity. While all the answer choices are common measurements of airflow, the more sensitive measure to diagnose COPD is the FEV_1:FVC ratio. It is considered normal if it is 70% or more of the predicted value based on the patient's gender, age, and height. The TLC is not often used in the routine management of COPD, but may be important for restrictive disease.

391. The answer is b. (*South-Paul, pp 380-391.*) Of the 300,000 patients in the United States with end-stage renal disease (ESRD), one-third of those have their disease because of diabetic nephropathy. While the other listed answers may cause ESRD, diabetes is the most common cause.

392. The answer is d. (*Rakel, pp 882-889.*) Weight, diabetes, and hypertension, by themselves, do not indicate the presence or absence of renal insufficiency. However, most cases of chronic renal failure are caused by diabetes and hypertension (60%), so those should be recognized as significant risk factors. The serum creatinine level can be normal in elderly people with chronic renal insufficiency, because they generally have less muscle mass. Therefore, the best indicator of the presence of renal failure is the GFR. The other tests mentioned are not sufficient tests, and normal values in these tests do not indicate that the patient does not have renal insufficiency.

393. The answer is e. *(Rakel, pp 882-889.)* The kidney's role in concentrating and diluting urine is usually retained until the GFR falls below 30% of normal. Therefore, hyponatremia, hyperkalemia, hyperphosphatemia, and metabolic acidosis (because of a fall in plasma bicarbonate) generally occur in later stages of kidney disease. The kidney is the source of erythropoietin, and anemia generally appears when the GFR falls below 60 mL/min.

394. The answer is c. *(Rakel, pp 882-889.)* The National Kidney Foundation ← staging system is useful to clinicians as it helps guide appropriate testing and referral for patients with kidney failure. Stage 0 represents people at risk for renal failure, but with a GFR greater than 90 mL/min. In these people, control of blood pressure and diabetes may forestall the progression to kidney failure. Stage 1 renal failure represents evidence of renal damage (either microalbuminuria or proteinuria), but with a GFR greater than 90 mL/min. Stage 2 renal failure represents mildly reduced GFR (values between 60-90 mL/min). In stage 3, the GFR is between 30 to 59 mL/min. Stage 4 represents moderate to severe renal failure with GFR levels from 15 to 29 mL/min, and stage 5 represents severe renal failure with GFR less than 15 mL/min.

395. The answer is d. *(Rakel, pp 882-889.)* According to National Kidney Foundation guidelines, this patient has stage 1 renal failure. ACE inhibitors should be added to his regimen to prevent the evolution of microalbuminuria to full blown proteinuria. Improvements in diet and exercise are always appropriate, but should not take the place of the addition of an ACE inhibitor. Checking a glycosolated hemoglobin level would not be indicated as a screen for diabetes.

396. The answer is d. *(Rakel, pp 882-889.)* The patient's laboratory values and clinical picture is consistent with moderate renal failure (National Kidney Foundation stage 3). At this point, nephrology referral is indicated. Renal replacement therapy (transplant or dialysis) is indicated for severe renal insufficiency (GFR less than 15 mL/min).

397. The answer is e. *(Goldberg, 2006.)* Liver tests are followed in patients with cirrhosis to assess severity and progress. While all of the tests above may be abnormal in patients with cirrhosis, bilirubin may be normal if the cirrhosis is well-compensated. Rising serum bilirubin may indicate a poor prognosis in patients with primary biliary cirrhosis.

398. The answer is a. (*Goldberg, 2006.*) Hyponatremia is common in patients with cirrhosis and ascites and is related to the inability to excrete free water. This results from high levels of antidiuretic hormone secretion.

399. The answer is e. (*Goldberg, 2006.*) The gold standard for diagnosing cirrhosis is the examination of the liver following transplantation or autopsy. In clinical practice, cirrhosis is diagnosed with a liver biopsy. The sensitivity of liver biopsy is in between 80% to 100%. Biopsy is not necessary if the clinical, laboratory, and radiologic data strongly suggest the presence of cirrhosis. This may be the case in a patient with ascites, coagulopathy, and a shrunken nodular appearing liver on ultrasound.

400. The answer is e. (*Goldberg, 2006.*) Determining the cause of liver disease has important implications for treatment. The most important aspect of diagnosing alcoholic liver disease is the documentation of chronic alcohol abuse. However, alcohol use is sometimes denied by the patient. Alcoholic hepatitis is associated with the classic laboratory findings of a disproportionate elevation of AST compared to ALT with both values usually being less than 300 IU/L. This ratio is generally greater than 2.0, a value rarely seen in other forms of liver disease, including those listed in this question (viral or autoimmune hepatitis or hematochromatosis).

401. The answer is e. (*Mengel, pp 442-447.*) Laboratory studies that represent acute hepatocellular injury include AST, ALT, LDH, and alkaline phosphatase. Laboratory values that represent hepatic function include albumin, bilirubin, and prothrombin time. Tests of hepatic function are more suggestive of chronic disease as opposed to acute injury.

402. The answer is c. (*Mengel, pp 442-447.*) Varicies occur secondary to chronic high pressure in the portal veins. Bleeding from varicies is the most common cause of death in the cirrhotic patients. The other potential causes of death listed are less common.

403. The answer is b. (*Mengel, pp 442-447.*) Absolute contraindications to liver transplantation include portal vein thrombosis, severe medical illness, malignancy, hepatobiliary sepsis, or lack of patient understanding. Relative contraindications are active alcoholism, HIV or hepatitis B surface antigen positivity, extensive previous abdominal surgery, and a lack of a personal support system.

404. The answer is c. *(Mengel, pp 447-458.)* BNP is elevated in both systolic and diastolic heart failure, and is helpful for distinguishing heart failure from other causes of dyspnea. Wheezes are common with heart failure, as bronchospasm may occur as a consequence of transudate into the alveoli and mucosal congestion. Dullness to percussion occurs with pulmonary edema. A pulmonary embolus may present with an elevated BNP, but a deep venous thrombosis would likely not involve both legs and cause bilateral lower extremity edema. Aspiration would not lead to an increased BNP.

405. The answer is a. *(Mengel, pp 447-458.)* Routine laboratory testing in a person with the new diagnosis of heart failure includes an electrocardiogram, a CBC, a urinalysis, serum creatinine, potassium and albumin levels, and thyroid function studies. An echocardiogram is imperative to help identify structural abnormalities of the heart and to measure the ejection fraction. Holter monitoring is not routinely warranted, as it would not identify a cause for heart failure, but would be used to identify an arrhythmia. Catheterization or stress testing may be important if ischemia or ischemic cardiomyopathy is identified as a cause, but is not a routine initial test.

406. The answer is b. *(Mengel, pp 447-458.)* The NYHA functional classification is important for clinicians to understand, as therapy may change as patients progress from class to class. Class I patients have no limitation of activity. Class II patients have slight limitations, are comfortable at rest, but have fatigue, palpitations, dyspnea, or angina with ordinary activity. Class III patients are also comfortable at rest, but less than ordinary activity causes symptoms. Class IV patients have symptoms at rest, and increased symptoms with even minor activity. There is no "class V" in this system.

407. The answer is e. *(Mengel, pp 447-458.)* Many noncardiac comorbid conditions may affect the proper diagnosis and clinical course of heart failure. All of the interventions in this question should be done, but only discontinuing alcohol use has actually been shown to improve function significantly. Optimally treating COPD is important, as exacerbations from heart failure are often difficult to distinguish from COPD exacerbations. Optimally treating diabetes and hypertension will minimize the negative effects of these conditions on the heart, but will not improve damage already done. Cigarette smoking should be discontinued, but generally does not lead to functional improvement.

Those with alcoholic cardiomyopathy actually see improvement of the left ventricular function with abstinence.

408. The answer is a. (*Mengel, pp 447-458.*) Many clinical trials have shown that ACE inhibitors decrease symptoms, improve quality of life, decrease hospitalizations, and reduce mortality in patients with NYHA class II to IV heart failure. In addition, they slow the progression to heart failure among asymptomatic patients with left ventricular systolic dysfunction. All patients with heart failure should be prescribed an ACE inhibitor unless they have a contraindication. β-Blockers are helpful, but not necessarily as a first-line agent. Nitrates and hydralazine can be used in patients who do not tolerate ACE inhibitors, as can ARBs. Some calcium channel blockers (nifedipine, diltiazem, and nicardipine) may worsen systolic dysfunction.

409. The answer is d. (*Mengel, pp 447-458.*) Some patients have difficulty maintaining optimal fluid balance, and a second diuretic is needed. In this case, adding metolazone can significantly increase diuresis in the out-patient treatment of heart failure with volume overload. Prolonged therapy should be avoided. Hydrocholorozide would not enhance diuresis, nor would triamterene. Spironolactone can be used, but is usually only considered for NYHA class III or IV patients or those with a serum potassium level less than 5.0 mmol/L.

410. The answer is c. (*McPhee, pp 341-351.*) ACE inhibitors and ARBs do not have the same effects on the neurohormonal pathways involved in CHF. However the valsartan in heart failure trial showed that while valsartin (an ARB) added to an ACE inhibitor decreases hospitalization in patients with CHF, it did not decrease mortality. The Candesartan in Heart Failure: Assessment of Reduction in Mortality and Morbidity (CHARM) trial showed that rates of cardiovascular death and heart failure admissions were similar in patients with CHF that were treated with ACE inhibitors or ARBs.

411. The answer is c. (*Mengel, pp 447-458.*) β-Blockers inhibit the adverse effects of sympathetic nervous system activation in heart failure patients. Studies have shown that three β-blockers (bisoprolol, metoprolol, and carvedilol) can reduce symptoms, improve quality of life and reduce mortality. Adding diuretics does not change mortality. Nifedipine can worsen symptoms. Digoxin improves symptoms, but does not decrease mortality.

412. The answer is e. *(Rakel, pp 1071-1077.)* Loss of synapses is believed to be the critical pathologic substrate of Alzheimer disease. Brain atrophy, destruction of neurons, and shrinkage of neurons occur commonly in the disease, but are also seen in elderly patients without the disease.

413. The answer is b. *(Rakel, pp 1071-1077.)* The decline in cholinergic activity associated with Alzheimer is well-documented, and is the basis for the approved treatments for the disease. Additional changes have been noted, including deficiencies in glutamate, norepinephrine, serotonin, somatostatin, and corticotropin-releasing factors, but these are less consistent.

414. The answer is d. *(Rakel, pp 1071-1077.)* Dementia is often difficult to distinguish from delirium or depression in the elderly. However, delirium is generally acute in onset and associated with a loss of concentration. Dementia's onset is insidious, and concentration is less likely to be a problem. Depression is associated with psychomotor slowing, while dementia is generally not. While people with dementia may complain of memory loss, it is far more likely that the patient's family will complain of the patient having memory loss in dementia. Depressed patients usually present themselves complaining of memory loss. Depressed and delirious patients will generally show poor effort in testing, while demented patients will generally display good effort, but get wrong answers.

415. The answer is e. *(Rakel, pp 1071-1077.)* Often, memory disturbances are the presenting symptom in Alzheimer's disease. Remote memories are well-preserved initially, with the ability to recall new information being lost early in the illness. Decreased conversational output is also noted early. Decreased ability to recognize and draw complex figures is an early sign of problems, as is the loss of the ability to calculate. Social propriety and interpersonal skills often remain strikingly preserved until late in the illness.

416. The answer is d. *(Rakel, pp 1071-1077.)* In the past, it was thought that vascular dementia (multi-infarct dementia, or that occurring after a stroke) was common. This is because MRI scans from demented patients often show changes consistent with small-vessel ischemic disease. Those changes are not seen as being significant without the appropriate clinical picture. The typical history would include episodic abrupt changes, as described in this question, and imaging findings consistent with ischemia. Alzheimer disease, Parkinson disease, and alcoholic dementia would likely be more insidious in onset. Depression is often a problem in the elderly, and may be mistaken for dementia. It would not follow the described course, however.

417. The answer is c. *(Rakel, pp 1071-1077.)* Three cholinesterase inhibitors are approved for the treatment of Alzheimer disease. They include donepezil (Aricept), galantamine (Reminyl), and rivastigmine (Exelon). They reduce the metabolism of acetylcholinesterase, thereby prolonging its action at cholinergic synapses. They are associated with modest improvements in cognition, behavior, activities of daily living and global measurements of functioning. However, they do not change the progression of neurodegeneration.

418. The answer is d. *(Rakel, pp 1071-1077. Mengel, pp 459-476.)* The patient described has dementia of Lewy body (DLB) type. This begins similarly to Alzheimer disease, but then patients develop complex visual hallucinations and spontaneous signs of parkinsonism. Patients with Alzheimer dementia develop delusions, but rarely have hallucinations. Antipsychotics should be avoided in this type of dementia, unless absolutely necessary, as there is concern for long-term neurological damage. DLB responds to cholinesterase inhibitors, and the other medications listed are safe if used appropriately.

419. The answer is d. *(McPhee, pp 56-59.)* Evidence from clinical trials has shown that donepezil can result in modest clinical improvement versus placebo in community-dwelling patients with dementia, but found no difference in the rates of institutionalization or progression of disease. Patients with more advanced disease have been shown to have statistically significant benefit from Memantine, with or without concomitant use of an acetylcholinesterase inhibitor. Ginkgo biloba has been shown to have mixed results in studies.

420. The answer is b. *(South-Paul, pp 380-391.)* The American Diabetes Association recommends screening all persons older than 45 years for diabetes every 3 years. Screens should start earlier in people with risk factors including a family history of diabetes in a first-degree relative, hypertension, obesity, high-risk ethnic groups (African American, Hispanic, Native American), a previous history of impaired glucose tolerance, abnormal lipids (especially elevated triglycerides and low HDL), and women with a history of gestational diabetes or a birth of a child greater than 9 lb. Multiple screens are available. Random glucose is easy, but has low specificity. A 2-hour glucose tolerance test is more specific, but is more costly and time consuming. A 1-hour glucose tolerance test is generally used for screening pregnant women, with a 3-hour glucose tolerance test being used for those that are positive. Urinalyses are highly specific, but have low sensitivity. Fasting glucose is more accurate, and is generally recommended.

421. The answer is c. *(South-Paul, pp 380-391.)* The diagnosis of diabetes may be made by two separate random glucose measurements more than 200 mg/dL with classic signs of diabetes (polydipsia, polyuria, polyphagia, weight loss), a fasting glucose greater than 126 mg/dL, or a glucose reading greater than 200 mg/dL 2 hours after a 75-g glucose load.

422. The answer is a. *(South-Paul, pp 380-391.)* In the past, young adults diagnosed with diabetes were primarily type 1. However, the epidemic of obesity in the United States has increased the rate of type 2 diabetes in people less than 20 years old from 5% to 30% over the last decade. C-peptide is cleaved from natively produced insulin. In people with type 1 diabetes, C-peptide levels should be low. Microalbuminuria, markedly elevated hemoglobin A1C and peripheral neuropathy can all occur in type 1 or 2 diabetes.

423. The answer is d. *(South-Paul, pp 380-391.)* The first indication of renal compromise in diabetics is an increase in GFR. Renal lesions develop, and are followed by microalbuminuria. Uncorrected, this can lead to macroalbuminuria, then renal failure. ACE inhibitors have been shown to decrease end-stage renal disease and death by 41% in diabetics. Lifestyle changes including glucose control, weight loss, and decreased protein intake can help, but experts agree that the benefits of ACE inhibitors are well-documented. Nephrology referral would be indicated if the creatinine becomes elevated, or in the face of macroalbuminuria or microalbuminuria despite maximal therapy. Even in patients who are normotensive, low-dose ACE inhibitors are beneficial in the face of microalbuminuria.

424. The answer is a. *(South-Paul, pp 380-391.)* Diabetic retinopathy is the leading cause of blindness in the United States. The risk increases with the length of time that the patient has had diabetes, and the condition worsens with increasing hemoglobin A1C levels. In type 2 diabetics, it can be seen at diagnosis. Aspirin has no effect on eye complications. It follows a predictable pattern, with mild background abnormalities followed by increased vascular permeability and hemorrhage. Proliferative changes occur late in the course.

425. The answer is c. (*South-Paul, pp 380-391.*) ACE inhibitors are clearly the first choice for blood pressure control in diabetic patients. They control blood pressure effectively, help prevent progression of renal disease, and are indicated in the presence of coronary disease and CHF. The other listed medications can be added for improved control if needed.

426. The answer is b. (*South-Paul, pp 380-391.*) Statins are the drug of choice in treating hyperlipidemia in diabetes. They have been shown to decrease the risk of coronary events and are excellent in lowering LDL. They do have less effect on the triglyceride levels, but in many patients, the decrease is enough to get patients to goal. Niacin will decrease triglycerides, raise HDL, and lower LDL, but may increase insulin resistance. Niacin is often used in combination with a statin or alone in patients with statin side-effects. Fibric acid derivatives lower triglycerides and raise HDL, but have minimal effects on LDL. Bile acid resins sequester bile acids in the GI tract. They can increase triglyceride levels, and are generally not used in diabetics.

427. The answer is a. (*South-Paul, pp 380-391.*) Glycemic control is dependent on the total caloric intake, not the type of calorie taken in. Low-carbohydrate and high-protein diets have not been shown to improve glucose control more than weight loss from other methods. Sucrose does not need to be eliminated, but it may raise blood sugar more quickly after ingestion. Formal dietary programs are not more likely to produce long-term sustainable results unless exercise is a large component of the plan. Increased fiber does improve glycemic control.

428. The answer is d. (*South-Paul, pp 380-391.*) Oral therapy for type 2 diabetes can be complicated. No evidence supports changing sulfonylureas when one isn't adequately controlling glucose levels. Biguanides act to decrease glucose output from the liver, and can decrease hemoglobin A1C by 1.5% to 2%. However, biguanides should not be used if creatinine is higher than 1.5 mg/dL. Meglitinides increase insulin secretion, and should only be taken before meals. They can reduce the hemoglobin A1C by 0.5% to 2% and are most valuable if fasting sugar is adequate, but postprandial sugars are high. Since they increase insulin levels, they are more effective when used in combination with a medication that has a different mechanism of action. They are excreted in the liver, therefore are safe in renal failure. Thiazolidinediones decrease insulin resistance and are an excellent choice for those with insulin insensitivity. α-Glucosidase inhibitors inhibit the absorption of carbohydrates in the gut and can decrease the hemoglobin A1C by 0.7% to 1%. They should be avoided if creatinine more than 2.0 mg/dL.

429. The answer is d. *(Hinnen et al, pp 612-620.)* The recently approved incretin-mimetic agent exenatide is indicated for patients who have not achieved adequate glycemic control with oral agents that include metformin and sulfonylureas. Studies with thiazolidinediones are forthcoming. Patients taking exenatide experience modest reductions in weight and in HbA$_{1C}$. Incretinmimetic agents have multiple mechanisms of action for the treatment of type 2 diabetes mellitus, including enhancement of glucose-dependent insulin secretion, suppression of inappropriately elevated glucagon, slowing of gastric emptying, and decreased food intake.

430. The answer is b. *(MacFarlane and Fisher, pp 297-304.)* Thiazolidinediones have been associated with an increased risk of peripheral edema. A meta-analysis was performed to assess the overall risk for developing edema secondary to thiazolidinediones. Odds ratios were generated by pooling estimates across the studies. The pooled odds ratio for thiazolidinediones induced edema was 2.26 (95% CI: 2.02-2.53). The results yielded a higher risk for developing edema with rosiglitazone (3.75 [2.70-5.20]) compared to pioglitazone (2.42 [1.90-3.08]). This meta-analysis demonstrates at least a twofold increase in the risk for developing edema with a thiazolidinediones agent. The risk appears to be greater with rosiglitazone than with pioglitazone.

Despite an increase in fluid-related events, recent studies suggest that individuals with type 2 diabetes mellitus and heart failure (New York Heart Association grade I/II) can be treated with thiazolidinediones with appropriate monitoring and adjustment of heart failure therapies.

431. The answer is e. *(Drucker, pp 1696-1705.)* Glucagon-like peptide 1 (GLP-1) is a gut-derived incretin hormone that stimulates insulin and suppresses glucagon secretion, inhibits gastric emptying, and reduces appetite and food intake. Therapeutic approaches for enhancing incretin action include degradation-resistant GLP-1 receptor agonists (incretin mimetics), and inhibitors of dipeptidyl peptidase-4 (DPP-4) activity (incretin enhancers). Orally administered DPP-4 inhibitors, such as sitagliptin reduce HbA$_{1C}$ by 0.5% to 1.0%, with few adverse events and no weight gain. These new classes of antidiabetic agents, and incretin mimetics and enhancers, also expand β-cell mass in preclinical studies.

432. The answer is a. *(Mengel, pp 476-484.)* It is important to thoroughly understand the action of the different types of insulin preparations in order to make therapeutic decisions about diabetic patients and their control. Aspart has the most rapid onset of action, between 15 to 30 minutes. Regular insulin has an onset between 30 to 60 minutes. Lente's onset is between 1 to 2 hours, as is Lantus'. Ultralente's onset is between 2 to 4 hours.

433. The answer is c. (*Mengel, pp 476-484.*) It is important to thoroughly understand the action of the different types of insulin preparations in order to make therapeutic decisions about diabetic patients and their control. Aspart's activity peaks early, between 30 to 60 minutes after injection. Regular insulin peaks between 2 to 3 hours after injection. Lente's peak is between 4 to 8 hours, and Ultralente's peak is between 8 to 20 hours. One of the important things to remember about Lantus is that it does not have a peak.

434. The answer is d. (*Mengel, pp 476-484.*) It is important to thoroughly understand the action of the different types of insulin preparations in order to make therapeutic decisions about diabetic patients and their control. Aspart's duration of action is between 3 to 5 hours. Regular insulin lasts between 4 to 12 hours. Lente's duration is between 10 to 20 hours, and Lantus' duration is around 24 hours. The longest duration is with Ultralente, which lasts 24 to 32 hours.

435. The answer is c. (*Mengel, pp 476-484.*) There are many methods for determining the appropriate amount of insulin that will be required in type 1 diabetics. One way is to determine the total amount of insulin used while hospitalized, and divide that dose during the day. Two-thirds of the total insulin should be given in the morning, with the remaining one-third in the evening. Each time the patient receives insulin, 75% of the dose should be NPH, and 25% should be regular. In this question, the patient needed 100 U of insulin. Of this, 67 U should be given in the morning, and 33 U should be given in the evening. Of the morning dose, 75% should be NPH. Seventy-five percent of 67 U equals to 50 U. Therefore, the patient should get 50 U of NPH in the morning and 17 U of regular.

436. The answer is c. (*Mengel, pp 476-484.*) When using Lantus and Lispro, approximately 40% to 50% of the total daily insulin requirements should be given as Lantus, with the remaining 50% to 60% of insulin given as Lispro before each meal, based on a preprandial glucose reading.

437. The answer is b. (*Mengel, pp 476-484.*) Patients with type 2 diabetes may require insulin therapy if diet, exercise, and oral hypoglycemic agent do not provide appropriate control. A low dose of NPH is commonly used, estimating 0.1 U/kg of body weight, as an addition to the current regimen.

438. The answer is b. *(Koski, pp 869-876.)* Metformin should be withheld before a procedure with radiocontrast dye, as contrast-induced nephropathy may predispose to developing lactic acidosis if a patient is taking concurrent metformin. It should also be withheld for surgery. It can be restarted immediately after surgery if the person's renal function is normal and his or her condition is stable.

439. The answer is a. *(Mengel, pp 484-499.)* Alcohol, in moderation, raises HDL cholesterol. Alternatively, cigarette smoking decreases HDL. Being overweight or obese decreases HDL, but weight loss may not raise HDL. Low dietary intake of cholesterol or high dietary intake of protein has not been shown to impact HDL. Stress can markedly increase LDL cholesterol, but will not impact HDL.

440. The answer is a. *(Mengel, pp 484-499.)* Blood lipids change acutely in response to food intake. The triglyceride level is lowest in the fasting state, and rises by an average of 50 mg/dL postprandially. As the triglyceride level rises, the total and LDL cholesterol each fall. Thus total and LDL cholesterol tend to be higher when fasting. HDL varies little whether fasting or not.

441. The answer is c. *(Mengel, pp 484-499.)* Of all the lipid values, low HDL is the single best predictor of an adverse outcome. However, high HDL does not guarantee immunity from coronary artery disease. C-reactive protein levels predict risk for myocardial infarction and stroke even better than LDL levels do, but are not as beneficial as HDL.

442. The answer is d. *(Mengel, pp 484-499.)* Smoking cessation increases HDL by 5 to 10 mg/dL, but does not affect LDL, VLDL, or triglycerides.

443. The answer is d. *(Mengel, pp 484-499.)* Aspirin blocks much of the flushing that is associated with sustained-release niacin preparations. Taking niacin at night, with food, on an empty stomach or with milk, or with a proton pump inhibitor will not impact the side effects.

444. The answer is e. *(McPhee, pp 1074-1084. Mengel, pp 484-499.)* Pravastatin (Pravachol), fluvastatin (Lescol), and rosuvastatin (Crestor) are not metabolized by the cytochrome P-450 3A4 enzyme system and therefore have less potential for drug interactions. Atorvastatin (Lipitor), simvastatin (Zocor), lovastatin (Mevacor) either alone or in combination are more likely to cause interactions. Pravastatin can be expected to lower LDL by 25% to 40% and increase HDL by 5% to 10%. Rosuvastatin can be expected to decrease LDL by 40% to 50% and increase HDL by 10% to 15%.

445. The answer is e. *(Mengel, pp 484-499.)* Fish oil is high in omega-3 fatty acids and have been shown to be beneficial in lowering cholesterol. Fish oils work by decreasing secretion of triglycerides by the liver.

446. The answer is b. *(Mengel, pp 484-499.)* Gemfibrozil changes the hepatic metabolism of lipoproteins and is a logical choice for the patient with low HDL and elevated triglycerides.

447. The answer is d. *(Mengel, pp 484-499.)* Ezetemibe (Zetia) lowers cholesterol by interfering with the absorption of cholesterol in the gut. Used alone, it lowers LDL and triglycerides only modestly. When added to a low-dose statin, the combination lowers LDL as much as the maximum statin dose, but its combined use with a low-dose statin may produce fewer adverse effects.

448. The answer is d. *(McPhee, pp 1074-1084.)* The different options for medical management of hyperlipidemia include preparations that affect the total cholesterol, the HDL, the LDL, and the triglycerides. Choice of medication depends on the desired endpoint. The following table outlines the expected increase in HDL that would be expected using the medications in the answer key:

Medication	Increase in HDL
Lovastatin	5%-10%
Colestipol	Approximately 5%
Ezetimibe	Approximately 5%
Fenofibrate	15%-25%
Cholestyramine	Approximately 5%

Niacin is even better than fenofibrate, increasing HDL by 25% to 35% on average.

449. The answer is a. (*McPhee, pp 1074-1084.*) The following table outlines the expected decrease in LDL that would be expected using the medications in the answer key:

Medication	Increase in HDL
Lovastatin	25%-40%
Colestipol	15%-25%
Ezetimibe	Approximately 20%
Fenofibrate	10%-15%
Cholestyramine	15-25%

The best statin for decreasing LDL is rosuvastatin. It can lower LDL by 40% to 50%.

450. The answer is d. (*McPhee, pp 1074-1084.*) The following table outlines the expected decrease in triglycerides that would be expected using the medications in the answer key:

Medication	Decrease in TG
Lovastatin	Mild
Colestipol	No effect
Ezetimibe	No effect
Fenofibrate	Moderate
Cholestyramine	No effect

Fenofibrate can be expected to decrease triglycerides by approximately 40%.

451. The answer is b. (*McPhee, pp 1074-1084.*) Niacin was the first lipid-lowering agent associated with decreased total mortality. It moderately decreases LDL, can increase HDL by 20% to 25%, and moderately decreases triglycerides. It causes a prostaglandin-mediated flushing that patients often describe as "hot flashes." This side effect can be easily moderated by having the patient take a NSAID or aspirin at least an hour before taking the niacin. Although niacin can increase blood sugar, it is safe for diabetics to use.

452. The answer is e. (*McPhee, pp 1150-1177.*) Postexposure prophylaxis against HIV can substantially decrease the risk of seroconversion after a needle stick injury. Healthcare workers should be tested for HIV as soon as possible after the needle stick to establish a negative baseline for potential worker's compensation claim, should the worker subsequently seroconvert. Therapy should be initiated using at least two medications to which the source would unlikely be resistant. Some clinicians prefer triple therapy.

453. The answer is d. (*McPhee, pp 1150-1177.*) Testing to establish the diagnosis of HIV infection usually requires an ELISA followed by a confirmatory Western blot of immunofluorescent antibody test. However, there is a "window period" of several weeks to 3 months between the infection and seroconversion when these tests may be negative. During this time, patients may be viremic and infectious, but not have sufficient levels of antibodies to result in positive tests. If there is strong clinical suspicion, plasma HIV RNA should be ordered. This, however, also needs to be interpreted with caution, as low level viremia may represent a false-positive test. CD4 count is not helpful in acute HIV disease.

454. The answer is a. (*McPhee, pp 1150-1177.*) The incidence of cervical dysplasia in HIV positive women is 40%. More HIV infected women die of cervical cancer than do from AIDS, therefore Pap testing should be done every 6 months. Some recommend routine colposcopy regardless of the Pap results. Cone biopsy should be reserved for cases of serious dysplasia.

455. The answer is c. (*McPhee, pp 1150-1177.*) Usually, induration of 15 mm (10 mm in high-risk patients) indicates a positive test. In HIV-infected individuals, 5 mm is considered a positive test. PPD tests should be placed annually in HIV-infected patients, as there is an increased risk of progression from latent to active TB in infected individuals.

456. The answer is a. (*McPhee, pp 1150-1177.*) Prophylaxis against *M avium* complex (MAC) should be instituted once the patient's CD4 count drops below 75 to 100 lymphocytes/mm^3. Prophylaxis against *Pneumocystis* pneumonia should be considered once the CD4 count drops below 200 lymphocytes/mm^3. Prophylaxis for fungal disease has been studied, but there was no benefit in the group that had prophylaxis with regard to mortality. Prophylaxis for herpes simplex and herpes zoster is not generally done. CMV prophylaxis can be instituted in those with CMV IgG positivity and with CD4 counts below 50 lymphocytes/mm^3, but it is generally not done because ganciclovir (the primary prophylactic agent) can cause neutropenia.

457. The answer is c. (*McPhee, pp 1150-1177.*) The x-ray shown is suspicious for *Pneumocystis* pneumonia, and treatment should be started immediately. The treatment of choice is trimethoprim-sulfamethoxazole (TMP-SMX) for 3 weeks. However, if the Pao$_2$ is below 70 mm Hg, the patient should receive concurrent steroids.

458. The answer is a. (*McPhee, pp 1150-1177.*) HIV-drug resistance has been documented for all available antiretroviral medications, and exists even among drug-naïve patients who were infected with a resistant strain. Current expert guidelines recommend resistance testing for patients recently infected or newly diagnosed and for pregnant people. It is also recommended for patients on an antiretroviral regimen with suboptimal viral suppression.

459. The answer is e. (*Mengel, pp 499-507.*) The patient described above has stage 2 hypertension (systolic blood pressure greater or equal to 160 mm Hg, or diastolic blood pressure greater or equal to 90 mm Hg). Since lifestyle modifications have not helped, the next step is to institute drug therapy. JNC 7 guidelines state that in patients with stage 2 hypertension, two-drug combination therapy is indicated. The most common regimen would be a thiazide diuretic along with either an ACE inhibitor, ARB, β-blocker, or calcium channel blocker.

460. The answer is d. (*Mengel, pp 499-507.*) When examining a hypertensive patient, the physician should be alert for signs of end-organ damage and possible causes of secondary hypertension. Signs of end-organ damage include arteriolar narrowing, hemorrhages, exudates or papilledema, carotid bruits or jugular venous distension, a loud second heart sound or precordial heave, arrhythmias, absent peripheral pulses, and peripheral edema, just to name a few. Signs suggestive of secondary hypertension include abdominal or flank masses (polycystic kidneys), absence of femoral pulses (coarctation of the aorta), tachycardia/flushing/diaphoresis (pheochromocytoma), abdominal bruits (renal artery stenosis), pigmented striae (Cushing syndrome), or an enlarged thyroid gland (hyperthyroidism).

461. The answer is b. (*Mengel, pp 499-507.*) Baseline laboratory screening is important to assess for end-organ damage and identify patients at high risk for cardiovascular complications. The routine tests for a newly diagnosed hypertensive patient include: hemoglobin and hematocrit, potassium, creatinine, fasting glucose, calcium, a fasting lipid profile, urinalysis, and a resting electrocardiogram. Other tests are not indicated unless physical examination or history makes them likely to be positive.

462. The answer is b. (*Mengel, pp 499-507.*) The patient described in the question has physical examination findings consistent with renal artery stenosis. A captopril renal scan or renal magnetic resonance angiography would evaluate this. Urinary metanephrines and vanillymandelic acid levels would help rule out pheochromocytoma. A chest x-ray would be helpful if coarctation of the aorta were suspected. An aortic CT would help to or quantify an aortic aneurysm, and an echocardiogram would help to identify left ventricular hypertrophy or systolic dysfunction.

463. The answer is a. (*McPhee, pp 370-397. Mengel, pp 499-507.*) While all of the interventions listed in this question have the potential to lower systolic blood pressure, losing 10 kg of body weight can lower systolic blood pressure by 5 to 20 mm Hg. The DASH diet (described in the landmark study, Dietary App-roaches to Stop Hypertension) is high in fruits and vegetables, with a reduced content of saturated and total fat can lower systolic blood pressure by 8 to 14 mm Hg. Sodium restriction will lower blood pressure by 2 to 8 mm Hg. Regular aerobic activity is also beneficial, lowering blood pressure by 4 to 9 mm Hg, and limiting alcohol can lower systolic blood pressure by 2 to 4 mm Hg.

464. The answer is a. (*Mengel, pp 499-507.*) The Antihypertensive and lipid-lowering treatment to prevent heart attack trial (ALLHAT) study and a meta-analysis of more than 42 clinical trials has demonstrated that low-dose diuretics are the most effective first-line treatment for preventing the occurrence of cardiovascular morbidity and mortality. If there are no compelling reasons to start another medication, it should be the medication of first choice.

465. The answer is c. (*Mengel, pp 499-507.*) The PROGRESS study (Perindopril Protection against Recurrent Stroke Study) found that an ACE inhibitor and diuretic in combination are effective in preventing recurrent stroke.

466. The answer is b. *(Mengel, pp 499-507.)* Several clinical trials have documented the benefit of ACE inhibitors in patients with hypertension and chronic kidney disease. Angiotension receptor blockers are also beneficial.

467. The answer is e. *(McPhee, pp 370-397.)* The British Hypertension Society developed recommendations to help practitioners devise an optimal treatment regimen when combining antihypertensives. They recommend that persons younger than 55 years who are not black start an ACE inhibitor as first-line therapy (A). β-Blockers (B) can be used in this group, but are no longer considered ideal first-line therapy. In persons older than 55 years or black, the first-line therapy is either a calcium channel blocker (C) or a diuretic (D). If one medication does not control the blood pressure, the next step is to add an agent from the other category. For example, if you have an "A" or "B" medication, add a "C" or "D" medication. If that still doesn't control the blood pressure, use A (or B) + C + D. Those still resistant should consider an α-blocker or other agent.

468. The answer is b. *(Mengel, pp 508-515.)* Atypical angina occurs when the patient experiences pain that has the quality and characteristics of angina, or occurs with exertion, but not both. For example, atypical angina may be a sense of heaviness not consistently related to exertion or relieved by rest, or it may be pain with an atypical character (sharp or stabbing) but predictably brought on by exercise and relieved by rest. Classic angina has both features. Anginal equivalent occurs when dyspnea is the sole or major manifestation. Nonanginal pain has neither the quality nor the precipitants of angina. "Atypical nonanginal pain" is not a term used to describe chest pain.

469. The answer is c. *(Mengel, pp 508-515.)* An anginal equivalent occurs when a patient has no chest pain, but has other symptoms of cardiac ischemia (eg, dyspnea) that is predictably precipitated by exertion and relieved by rest. Atypical angina occurs when the patient experiences pain that has the quality and characteristics of angina, or occurs with exertion, but not both. Nonanginal pain has neither the quality nor the precipitants of angina. "Atypical nonanginal pain" is not a term used to describe chest pain.

470. The answer is d. *(Mengel, pp 508-515.)* Nonanginal pain has neither the quality nor the precipitating features of angina. Typical descriptive terms of nonanginal pain include "stabbing," "shooting," "knifelike," "jabbing," and "tingling." Atypical angina occurs when the patient experiences pain that has the quality and characteristics of angina, or occurs with exertion, but not both. Anginal equivalent occurs when dyspnea is the sole or major manifestation. "Atypical nonanginal pain" is not a term used to describe chest pain.

471. The answer is b. (*Mengel, pp 508-515.*) The standard provocative test for ischemic heart disease is an exercise treadmill test. However, certain ECG abnormalities make the standard ETT unreadable. These include left ventricular hypertrophy with strain, left bundle branch block (shown in the question), and ST-segment baseline abnormalities in the precordial leads. In this case, a thallium ETT is preferred, as long as the patient can exercise.

472. The answer is d. (*Mengel, pp 508-515.*) Poor prognostic signs in an exercise treadmill test include failure to complete stage II of a Bruce protocol, failure to achieve a heart rate greater than 120 beats per minute (off β-blockers), onset of ST-segment depression at a heart rate less than 120 beats per minute, having ST-segment depression greater than 2.0 mm, having ST-segment depression lasting more than 6 minutes into recovery, poor systolic blood pressure response to exercise, angina or ventricular tachycardia with exercise, and ST-segment depression in multiple leads.

473. The answer is e. (*Mengel, pp 508-515.*) Tolerance is the most significant issue to consider when using nitrates for stable angina. Tolerance develops rapidly when long-acting nitrates are given. When using a patch, it is important to have intervals of 10 to 12 hours without the patch to retain the antianginal effect. Headache and fatigue may be important side effects, but are more of a nuisance than an important consideration. The medications can be used with β-blockers and calcium channel blockers.

474. The answer is c. (*Mengel, pp 508-515.*) All β-blockers, regardless of their selectivity, are equally effective in treating angina. About 20% of patients do not respond. The dose should be adjusted to achieve a heart rate of 50 to 60 beats per minute.

475. The answer is c. (*McPhee, pp 1086-1089.*) Current data estimates that 65% of Americans are overweight, and more than 35% are obese. Family physicians should be familiar with the use of BMI as an indicator of obesity and subsequent health risks. The BMI is determined by dividing the patient's weight in kilograms by the square of the height in meters. A BMI greater than 25 kg/m^2 is classified as overweight. A BMI greater than 30 kg/m^2 is considered obese, a BMI greater than 35 kg/m² is considered "class II obesity," and a BMI greater than 40 kg/m² is considered "class III obesity" or extreme obesity.

476. The answer is d. *(McPhee, pp 1086-1089.)* Unfortunately, only 20% of patients will lose 20 lb and maintain the weight loss for 2 years using conventional dietary techniques. Only 5% can maintain a 40 lb weight-loss. Those who are successful report continued close contact with their healthcare provider. Most successful programs are multidisciplinary and include a low-calorie diet, behavior modification, exercise, and social support.

477. The answer is a. *(McPhee, pp 1086-1089.)* The history and physical examination are of utmost importance when evaluating the obese patient. Less than 1% of obese patients have a secondary nonpsychiatric cause for their obesity. Hypothyroidism and Cushing syndrome are important examples that can generally be detected by history and physical (but would need additional testing if historical features or physical findings point in that direction). Laboratory evaluation is necessary, however, to assess the medical consequences of obesity, and include fasting glucose, LDL, HDL, and triglyceride levels.

478. The answer is d. *(McPhee, pp 1086-1089.)* Medications to treat obesity are available over the counter and by prescription. While controversy exists, the NIH clinical guidelines state that medications may be used as part of a comprehensive weight management plan. Appetite suppressants can be amphetamines (but those carry a significant risk for abuse) or nonamphetamine. Sibutramine (Meridia) is a prescription serotonin/norepinephrine blocker. There is a selective cannabinoid-1 receptor antagonist called rimonabant under investigation that looks promising, but future studies will help determine its place in the management of obesity. Orlistat blocks fat absorption from the GI tract.

479. The answer is b. *(McPhee, pp 1086-1089.)* Bariatric surgery is an increasingly more common treatment option for severe obesity. In the United States, the most common procedure performed is the Roux-en-Y gastric bypass. The procedure can result in substantial weight loss, up to 50% of the initial weight in some studies. Complications are common, and occur with about 40% of the cases. Operative mortality is actually quite low 0% to 1% in the first 30 days. Nutritional deficiencies are common postoperatively, and patients require life-long supplementation. Because of the risks of the surgery, bariatric surgery is limited to those with a BMI > 40 kg/m², or > 35 kg/m² if there are obesity-related comorbidities present.

480. The answer is d. (*South-Paul, pp 298-309.*) Osteoporosis is because of poor acquisition of bone mass or accelerated bone loss. African Americans are less at risk than Caucasians or Asians. There is no evidence that oral contraceptive use increases risk. Obesity is considered to be protective because of increased estrogen production, as long as the person is not sedentary. Hyperthyroidism is a common cause of accelerated bone loss. Breast-feeding is a significant drain on calcium stores, but studies have shown that the associated bone mineral loss is completely reversed within 12 months of weaning.

481. The answer is a. (*South-Paul, pp 298-309.*) Weight-bearing activity is known to retard bone loss. While there have been no randomized clinical trials comparing the effect of various activities on bone mass, recommended activities include walking, jogging, weight lifting, aerobics, stair climbing, field sports, racquet sports, court sports, and dancing. Swimming is questionable, as it is not weight-bearing. There is no data on cycling, skating, or skiing.

482. The answer is e. (*South-Paul, pp 298-309.*) Primary osteoporosis refers to deterioration of bone mass not associated with other chronic illnesses or problems. History and physical are neither sensitive enough nor sufficient for the diagnosis of primary osteoporosis. While decreased serum calcium may indicate malabsorption or a vitamin D deficiency, it is not useful as a diagnostic tool for osteoporosis. Measures of bone turnover, like serum human osteocalcin levels, are of research interest, but are not useful for screening. Imaging studies are best.

483. The answer is d. (*South-Paul, pp 298-309.*) Plain radiographs are not sensitive enough to diagnose osteoporosis until total density has decreased by 50%. Single and dual photon absorptiometry provide poor resolution and are less accurate than other methods. DEXA scanning is most precise and is the test of choice. Quantitative CT scanning is the most sensitive, but exposes patients to significant levels of radiation.

484. The answer is c. (*South-Paul, pp 298-309.*) Bone densitometry provides a T-score (the number of standard deviations above or below the mean matched to YOUNG controls) and a Z-score (the number of standard deviations above or below the mean-matched to age-matched controls). Z-scores are of little value to clinicians. A T-score more than 2.5 standard deviations below the mean (a score of −2.5 or lower) indicates osteoporosis.

485. The answer is b. (*South-Paul, pp 298-309.*) Absolute contraindications to estrogen-replacement therapy include a history of breast cancer or other estrogen-dependent cancer, undiagnosed or abnormal genital bleeding, and a history or an active thromboembolic disorder. Relative contraindications include migraine, a history of thromboembolism, familial hypertriglyceridemia, uterine leiomyoma, uterine cancer, gallbladder disease, a strong family history of breast cancer, chronic hepatic dysfunction, and endometriosis.

486. The answer is c. (*South-Paul, pp 298-309.*) Calcitonin directly inhibits osteoclastic bone resorption and is considered a reasonable treatment alternative for patients with established osteoporosis in whom estrogen-replacement therapy is not recommended. It has the unique characteristic of producing an analgesic effect with respect to bone pain and is often prescribed for patients who have suffered an acute osteoporotic fracture.

487. The answer is c. (*South-Paul, pp 298-309.*) Bisphosphonates work by binding to the bone surface and inhibiting osteoclastic activity. Vitamin D increases absorption of calcium in the GI tract. Estrogen and selective estrogen receptor modulators (raloxifene or Evista) work by blocking the activity of cytokines. Fluoride stimulates osteoblasts, but does not result in the formation of normal bone.

488. The answer is b. (*South-Paul, pp 577-584.*) Depression is commonly seen in primary care settings. In fact, it is estimated that only about 20% of depression-related healthcare occurs in mental healthcare settings. Nonpsychiatrists write approximately 80% of the prescriptions for antidepressants. Patients with major depressive disorder often present with vague physical symptoms rather than emotional complaints. To make the diagnosis of depression using *DSM* criteria, the patient must describe either depressed mood for most of the day nearly every day for at least 2 weeks, or loss of interest in usually enjoyable activities. Irritable mood may take the place of depressed mood to make the diagnosis as well. In addition to one of those two symptoms, the patient must experience other symptoms of depression, including sleep changes, feelings of guilt or worthlessness, loss of energy, loss of concentration, change in appetite, psychomotor speeding or slowing, or suicidal thoughts, plans, or intent.

489. The answer is b. (*McPhee, pp 897-902.*) The disorder described is posttraumatic stress disorder (PTSD)—a syndrome characterized by reexperiencing a traumatic event. Alcohol and drugs are commonly used by the patient to self-treat. Antidepressants are helpful to ameliorate the symptoms, with sertraline and paroxetine having FDA indications for treatment of this disorder. Alprazolam can be used, but there is significant concern for dependency problems. Sometimes antiepileptic medications can be used, but more studies are needed, and the FDA has not approved them for this disorder.

490. The answer is d. (*Mengel, pp 637-645.*) Physicians have various treatment options for depression. Studies have shown that the combination of medication and therapy offer the best treatment outcomes. However, antidepressants alone are effective in about 50% to 60% of patients with major depression. If a patient fails to respond to one medication, he or she may respond to another. At least 80% of patients with major depression will respond to at least one antidepressant medication. In order to prevent relapse, treatment should continue for 6 to 9 months. ECT has a high rate of therapeutic success, but is reserved for those who do not respond to other modalities of treatment.

491. The answer is e. (*Mengel, pp 637-645.*) While many of the newer antidepressants are well-tolerated, physicians should be familiar with the adverse effects and contraindications for their use. Nefazodone should not be used in patients with liver disease. Hypertension is a relative contraindication to venlafaxine. Patients experiencing hypersomnia and motor retardation should avoid nefazodone and mirtazapine. Patients who report agitation and insomnia should avoid bupropion and venlafaxine. Mirtazapine and tricyclic antidepressants are less preferred for patients with obesity. Bupropion is contraindicated for patients with seizure disorder.

492. The answer is a. (*South-Paul, pp 585-596. Mengel, pp 604-612.*) Anxiety disorders encompass several clinical conditions including generalized anxiety disorder, panic disorder, the phobias, obsessive-compulsive disorder, and posttraumatic stress disorder. Conversion disorder is not classified as an anxiety disorder, and involves an unintentionally produced motor or sensory function deficit, preceded by conflict or stress. Somatization disorder involves a history of many medical complaints for which treatment is sought that cannot be explained fully by a known medical condition, and is also not classified as an anxiety disorder. Anorexia is classified as an eating disorder, and histrionic personality disorder is a classified among the personality disorders, and involves a dramatic, attention-seeking, and emotional patient.

493. The answer is d. *(Mengel, pp 645-654.)* Eating disorders are psychological disorders in which the person afflicted has an altered perception of body weight or shape and disturbances of eating behavior. Distinguishing between anorexia and bulimia may be important from a treatment standpoint. Some characteristics are common to both eating disorders, while other characteristics may help to differentiate them. Both disorders involve self-evaluation that is unduly influenced by body weight and/or shape. While binge eating or purging are considered characteristics of bulimia, there is a binge eating/purging subtype of anorexia that involves that behavior as well. Both bulimics and binge eating/purging subtypes of anorexics may use diuretics, enemas, and laxatives. Both engage in inappropriate behaviors to prevent weight gain. However, bulimics sense a lack of control over eating during episodes of binging, while anorexics often feel a strong sense of control. This is a characteristic that may help distinguish the two.

494. The answer is a. *(McPhee, pp 919-931.)* In some bipolar patients, the diagnosis is made after the initiation of an antidepressant allows the patient to cycle into a manic phase. All the medications listed in this answer can be used to help bipolar disorder, but only the neuroleptics will be of benefit in the acute phase. Lithium, valproic acid, carbamazepine, and lamotrigine are all excellent options for maintenance once the acute mania is under control.

495. The answer is b. *(Mengel, pp 612-629.)* Of children diagnosed with ADHD, up to 60% will continue to exhibit symptoms into adulthood. In adults, symptoms of ADHD may be more subtle, and symptoms may actually change. Hyperactivity may be replaced with restlessness, and impulsivity may be replaced with inability to control emotions or social inappropriateness. Sleep and appetite disturbances in adults should alert the physician to the possibility of another disorder, especially depression.

496. The answer is c. *(Mengel, pp 612-629.)* Stimulants reduce symptoms of hyperactivity, impulsivity, and inattention. The mechanism of action is thought to be by inhibition of dopamine and norepinephrine reuptake. Approximately 70% of children respond to a specific stimulant, and 90% will respond to at least one stimulant. A positive response to stimulant medication is not diagnostic for ADHD. As children and adults without ADHD who take stimulants demonstrate improvement in attention, concentration, and memory tasks.

497. The answer is a. (*South-Paul, pp 392-402.*) The most common cause of thyroiditis is chronic lymphocytic thyroiditis (also called Hashimoto thyroiditis). It is the most common cause of goiter in the United States. Generally seen in middle-aged women, this generally presents with enlargement of the thyroid, and most often there is associated tenderness. Subacute lymphocytic thyroiditis is less common, and although an acute increase in thyroid size is seen, it is generally nontender. Subacute granulomatous thyroiditis usually follows a viral illness and is also associated with a mildly painful gland. Suppurative thyroiditis is rare, and is associated with fever, a swollen thyroid and clinical manifestations of a bacterial illness. Invasive fibrous thyroiditis presents as a gradually increasing gland that is firm, but is nontender.

498. The answer is a. (*South-Paul, pp 392-402.*) Primary hypothyroidism is common, usually a result of Hashimoto thyroiditis or after Graves disease. In this case, the TSH would be elevated, and the free T_3 and T_4 would be low. Secondary hypothyroidism is related to hypothalamic or pituitary dysfunction. Iodine deficiency is a cause of primary hypothyroidism. Subclinical hypothyroidism is when the TSH is elevated, but the T_3 and T_4 are normal. Thyroid resistance would present with the TSH, T_3, and T_4 all being elevated.

499. The answer is c. (*South-Paul, pp 392-402.*) Thyroid receptor antibodies are very specific, and differentiate Graves disease from other causes of hyperthyroidism. The TSH and free thyroid hormones are nonspecific, and only identify hyperthyroidism. Radionucleotide imaging is helpful in Graves, showing diffuse uptake, but is not necessarily specific. Thyroid ultrasonography can identify nodules, but is also a nonspecific test for differentiating causes of hyperthyroidism.

500. The answer is b. (*South-Paul, pp 392-402.*) Once a thyroid nodule is found, the next step in the workup is radionucleotide imaging. If a nodule takes up radiotracer, it is termed a "hot" nodule. Colloidal cysts and tumors do not take up tracer and are "cold" nodules. Therefore, "hot" nodules are more likely benign. Neurofibromas would also be "cold." Definitive diagnosis can be made through needle aspiration.

Bibliography

Books

Mahadevan SV, Garmel GM (eds). *An Introduction to Clinical Emergency Medicine.* New York, NY: Cambridge University Press; 2005.

McPhee SJ, Papadakis MA, Tierney LM (eds). *Current Medical Diagnosis & Treatment,* 47th ed. New York, NY: McGraw Hill; 2008.

Mengel MB, Schweibert LP (eds). *Family Medicine Ambulatory Care and Prevention.* 4th ed. New York, NY: Lange Medical Books/McGraw-Hill; 2005.

Rakel RE, Bope ET (eds). *Conn's Current Therapy 2006.* Philadelphia, PA: Saunders/Elsevier; 2006.

Rosner B. *Fundamentals of Biostatistics,* 6th ed. Pacific Grove, CA: Duxbury; 2006.

South-Paul JE, Matheny SC, Lewis EL (eds). *Current Diagnosis and Treatment in Family Medicine,* 2nd ed. New York, Lange Medical Books/McGraw-Hill, 2008.

Journal articles

Advisory Committee on Immunization Practices (ACIP). Recommended adult immunization schedule, United States, October 2007-September 2008. *MMWR.* 2007:56;Q1-Q4.

Advisory Committee on Immunization Practices. Updated recommendation from the Advisory Committee on Immunization Practices for use of 7-valent pneumococcal conjugate vaccine (PCV7) in children aged 24-59 months who are not completely vaccinated. *MMWR weekly.* April 4, 2008:57(13);343-344.

Advisory Committee on Immunization Practices. Recommended adult immunization schedule: United States, October 2007-September 2008. *Ann Intern Med.* 2007a;147:725-729.

Advisory Committee on Immunization Practices. Prevention of human papillomavirus infection: Provisional recommendations for immunization of girls and women with quadrivalent human papillomavirus vaccine. *Pediatrics.* 2007b;120:666-668.

Brennan T, Blank L, Cohen J, et al. Medical professionalism in the new millennium: A physician charter. *Ann Intern Med.* 2002;136:243-246.

Drucker DJ, Nauck MA. The incretin system: Glucagon-like peptide-1 receptor agonists and dipeptidyl peptidase-4 inhibitors in type 2 diabetes. *Lancet.* Nov 11, 2006;368(9548):1696-1705.

Hinnen D, Nielsen LL, Waninger A, et al. Incretin mimetics and DPP-IV inhibitors: New paradigms for the treatment of Type 2 diabetes. *J Am Board Fam Med.* 2006;19:612-620.

Koski RR. Practical review of oral antihyperglycemic agents for Type 2 diabetes mellitus. *Diabetes Educ.* 2006;32:869-876.

Lee C et al. Hepatitis B immunization for hepatitis B surface antigen positive-mothers. *Cochrane Database Syst Rev.* 2006;2:CD004790

MacFarlane DP, Fisher M. Thiazolidinediones in patients with diabetes mellitus and heart failure: Implications of emerging data. *Am J Cardiovasc Drugs.* 2006;6(5):297-304.

Websites

American Academy of Family Physicians, 2008. AAFP Summary of Recommendations for Clinical Preventive Services Tool. Available at http://www.aafp.org/online/en/home/clinical/exam.html. Accessed 12/15/2008.

Fletcher SW, Barton MB. Evaluation of breast lumps and abnormal mammograms. http://www.utdol.com/utd/content/topic.do?topicKey=genr_med/43947&type=A&selectedTitle=1~8. Accessed 8/27/06.

Goldberg E, Chopra S. Diagnostic approach to the patient with cirrhosis. http://www.utdol.com/utd/content/topic.do?topicKey=cirrhosi/6052&view=print. Accessed 11/28/2006.

Isaacs C, Fletcher SW, Peshkin BN. Genetic testing for breast and ovarian cancer. http://www.utdol.com/utd/content/topic.do?topicKen+breastcn/17177&view=print. Accessed 1/22/2008.

Light RW. Primary spontaneous pneumothorax in adults. http://www.utdol.com/utd/content/topic.do?topicKey=pleurdis/9228. Accessed 12/6/2006.

Mahutte NG, Duleba AJ. Evaluating diagnostic tests. http://www.utdol.com/utd/content/topic.do?topicKey=genr_med/28312&type=A&selectedTitle=1~5. Accessed 12/6/2006.

Meisel JL. Diagnostic approach to chest pain in adults. http://www.utdol.com/utd/content/topic.do?topicKey=pri_card/2346&type=A&selected Title=1~87. Accessed 12/6/2006.

The American Academy of Family Physicians. Recommendations for clinical preventative services. http://www.aafp.org/online/en/home/clinical/exam/ k-o.html. Accessed 10/03/2006.

Shadlen MF, Larson EB. Evaluation of cognitive impairment and dementia. http://www.utdol.com/utd/content/topic.do?topicKey=nuroegen/6698&type=A&selectedTitle=5~42. Accessed 2/25/2007.

Shammash JB, Kimmel SE, Morgan JP. Estimation of cardiac risk prior to non-cardiac surgery. http://www.utdol.com/utd/content/topic.do? topicKey=periart/7170&type=A&selectedTitle=6~58. Accessed 12/3/2006.

Smetana GW. Preoperative medical evaluation of the healthy patient. http://www.utdol.com/utd/content/topic.do?topicKey=med_cons/6474&view=print. Accessed 11/30/2006.

Swaroop VS, Chari ST. Clinical manifestations and diagnosis of acute pancreatitis. http://www.utdol.com/utd/content/topic.do?topicKey=pancdis/7667&type=A&selectedTitle=1~134. Accessed 12/7/2006.

Yeh S, Ward JI. Prevention of *Haemophilus influenzae* infection. http://www.uptodate.com/online/content/topic.do?topicKey=pedi_id/28804&selectedTitle=4~133&source=search_result. Accessed 3/17/2008.

Weller PF. Immunizations for travel. http://www.utdol.com/utd/content/topic.do?topidKey+immunize/6150&view=print. Accessed 11/30/2006.

Wolff K, Johnson RA, Suurmond D (eds). *Fitzpatrick's Color Atlas and Synopsis of Clinical Dermatology.* 5th ed. New York, McGraw-Hill; 2005.

Index

Notes